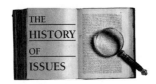

Mental Health

Other Books in the History of Issues Series:

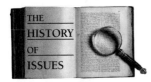

THE
HISTORY
OF
ISSUES

Mental Health

Adriane Ruggiero, Book Editor

GREENHAVEN PRESS

An imprint of Thomson Gale, a part of The Thomson Corporation

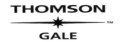

THOMSON

™

GALE

Detroit • New York • San Francisco • New Haven, Conn. • Waterville, Maine • London

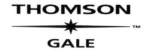

Christine Nasso, *Publisher*
Elizabeth Des Chenes, *Managing Editor*

© 2008 The Gale Group.

Star logo is a trademark and Gale and Greenhaven Press are registered trademarks used herein under license.

For more information, contact:
Greenhaven Press
27500 Drake Rd.
Farmington Hills, MI 48331-3535
Or you can visit our Internet site at http://www.gale.com

LIBRARY OF CONGRESS CATALOGING-IN-PUBLICATION DATA

Mental health / Adriane Ruggiero, book editor.
    p. cm. -- (History of issues)
    Includes bibliographical references and index.
    ISBN-13: 978-0-7377-3844-5 (hardcover)
    1. Mental health services--United States--History. 2. Mentally ill--Treatment--United States--History. 3. Psychiatry--United States--History. I. Ruggiero, Adriane.
    RA790.6.M366 2008
    362.2--dc22
                                                                2007024929

ISBN-10: 0-7377-3844-8 (hardcover)

Printed in the United States of America
10 9 8 7 6 5 4 3 2 1

Contents

Chapter 3: Revolutionary Changes Lead to the Modern Mental Health-Care System

Chapter 4: Mental Health Activism

Chapter 5: Improving Care for the Mentally Ill

Foreword

In the 1940s, at the height of the Holocaust, Jews struggled to create a nation of their own in Palestine, a region of the Middle East that at the time was controlled by Britain. The British had placed limits on Jewish immigration to Palestine, hampering efforts to provide refuge to Jews fleeing the Holocaust. In response to this and other British policies, an underground Jewish resistance group called Irgun began carrying out terrorist attacks against British targets in Palestine, including immigration, intelligence, and police offices. Most famously, the group bombed the King David Hotel in Jerusalem, the site of a British military headquarters. Although the British were warned well in advance of the attack, they failed to evacuate the building. As a result, ninety-one people were killed (including fifteen Jews) and forty-five were injured.

Early in the twentieth century, Ireland, which had long been under British rule, was split into two countries. The south, populated mostly by Catholics, eventually achieved independence and became the Republic of Ireland. Northern Ireland, mostly Protestant, remained under British control. Catholics in both the north and south opposed British control of the north, and the Irish Republican Army (IRA) sought unification of Ireland as an independent nation. In 1969, the IRA split into two factions. A new radical wing, the Provisional IRA, was created and soon undertook numerous terrorist bombings and killings throughout Northern Ireland, the Republic of Ireland, and even in England. One of its most notorious attacks was the 1974 bombing of a Birmingham, England, bar that killed nineteen people.

In the mid-1990s, an Islamic terrorist group called al Qaeda began carrying out terrorist attacks against American targets overseas. In communications to the media, the organization listed several complaints against the United States. It generally opposed all U.S. involvement and presence in the Middle East. It particularly objected to the presence of U.S. troops in Saudi Arabia, which is the home of several Islamic holy sites. And it strongly condemned the United States for supporting the nation of Israel, which it claimed was an oppressor of Muslims. In 1998 al Qaeda's leaders issued a fatwa (a religious legal statement) calling for Muslims to kill Americans. Al Qaeda acted on this order many times—most memorably on September 11, 2001, when it attacked the World Trade Center and the Pentagon, killing nearly three thousand people.

These three groups—Irgun, the Provisional IRA, and al Qaeda—have achieved varied results. Irgun's terror campaign contributed to Britain's decision to pull out of Palestine and to support the creation of Israel in 1948. The Provisional IRA's tactics kept pressure on the British, but they also alienated many would-be supporters of independence for Northern Ireland. Al Qaeda's attacks provoked a strong U.S. military response but did not lessen America's involvement in the Middle East nor weaken its support of Israel. Despite these different results, the means and goals of these groups were similar. Although they emerged in different parts of the world during different eras and in support of different causes, all three had one thing in common: They all used clandestine violence to undermine a government they deemed oppressive or illegitimate.

The destruction of oppressive governments is not the only goal of terrorism. For example, terror is also used to minimize dissent in totalitarian regimes and to promote extreme ideologies. However, throughout history the motivations of terrorists have been remarkably similar, proving the old adage that "the more things change, the more they remain the same." Arguments for and against terrorism thus boil down to the same set of universal arguments regardless of the age: Some argue that terrorism is justified to change (or, in the case of state terror, to maintain) the prevailing political order; others respond that terrorism is inhumane and unacceptable under any circumstances. These basic views transcend time and place.

Similar fundamental arguments apply to other controversial social issues. For instance, arguments over the death penalty have always featured competing views of justice. Scholars cite biblical texts to claim that a person who takes a life must forfeit his or her life, while others cite religious doctrine to support their view that only God can take a human life. These arguments have remained essentially the same throughout the centuries. Likewise, the debate over euthanasia has persisted throughout the history of Western civilization. Supporters argue that it is compassionate to end the suffering of the dying by hastening their impending death; opponents insist that it is society's duty to make the dying as comfortable as possible as death takes its natural course.

Greenhaven Press's The History of Issues series illustrates this constancy of arguments surrounding major social issues. Each volume in the series focuses on one issue—including terrorism, the death penalty, and euthanasia—and examines how the debates have both evolved and remained essentially the same over the years. Primary documents such as newspaper articles, speeches, and government reports illuminate historical developments and offer perspectives from throughout history. Secondary sources provide overviews and commentaries from a more contemporary perspective. An introduction begins each anthology and supplies essential context and background. An annotated table of contents, chronology, and index allow for easy reference, and a bibliography and list of organizations to contact point to additional sources of information on the book's topic. With these features, The History of Issues series permits readers to glimpse both the historical and contemporary dimensions of humanity's most pressing and controversial social issues.

Introduction

The psychological problems of returning Iraq War veterans are challenging the nation's mental health-care system and will continue to do so in the coming decades. While the physical risks of war may end when a soldier leaves the battlefield, experts in the mental health field believe the psychological toll of war continues to build, creating a mental health crisis with no end in sight.

Some of these war veterans, like veterans of earlier conflicts, show tremendous mental resilience and get on with their civilian lives with little trouble. Psychologists do not really know why this is; resilience could be a genetic component that some persons have and others do not. Many veterans lack this resilience, however, and are returning home with a wide array of mental ailments as result of their wartime experiences. While traumatic amputations, severe head wounds, and brain injuries are some of the most appalling physical injuries of the wars in Afghanistan and Iraq, many more vets suffer from anxiety and depression. In July 2004 a report published in the *New England Journal of Medicine* found that among soldiers who had returned from Iraq, one in six were suffering from symptoms of anxiety, depression, or post-traumatic stress disorder (PTSD).

Dr. Matthew Friedman, director of the Veterans Administration National Center, gave the following description of post-traumatic stress disorder: "PTSD is a recognition that if you've been in the wrong place at the wrong time or have been in a place where you've had to commit acts such as shooting other combatants or civilians or driven a car that you weren't in control of and killed people or things of that sort, that these events can change the way you feel about yourself and feel about the world. What's distinct about PTSD from almost all other psychiatric disorders is the fact that there is a historical event that sets this off. You had to be at Hiroshima; you had to be at Auschwitz; you had to be in Iraq; you had to be raped, mugged, in a plane crash or what have you. That, however, alone is not sufficient. Having been there, you also had to react to that situation with an extreme emotional reaction, what the American Psychiatric Association calls 'fear, helplessness or horror.'"[1]

A Mental Condition Old as War

Post-traumatic stress disorder is a relatively new name for a mental condition that is as old as war itself. Once called soldier's heart, shell shock, war exhaustion, or combat fatigue, PTSD was given its current name in the 1980s as society came to realize that the problems experienced by some Vietnam War (1965–1973) veterans were a distinct mental illness. The physical symptoms of PTSD include changes in blood pressure, heart rate, and pulse but these go away in time. It is the emotional effects that seem to be the longest lasting and the most debilitating. These include jumpiness, sleeplessness, anxiety, and a sense of emotional numbness and detachment. Many veterans describe themselves as being on pins and needles all the time. They may also experience vivid, unwanted memories or "flashbacks" of events they experienced. These events might be the deaths of fellow soldiers, the killing of civilians, or any random act of violence associated with war.

To some extent the anxiety, detachment, and flashbacks associated with PTSD seem to be normal responses to a traumatic event. These responses may even help some veterans come to terms with their trauma. The problem is that for some people, the condition continues for months or years after the trauma. It is these cases that mental health professionals consider to be PTSD.

Veterans who served in the Iraq War are especially prone to PTSD because soldiers in that war had a particularly high likelihood of being in combat. The nature of that combat further contributes to PTSD. The daily urban fighting, the suicide bombers, and the guerrilla tactics of insurgents who blend into the general public all create an extra layer of stress that takes its toll on a soldier, say psychologists Lynda King, PhD, and Daniel King, PhD, of the National Center for PTSD and the Massachusetts Veterans Epidemiology Research and Information Center.[2] A study of more than one hundred thousand veterans who have sought medical care since returning from war shows that nearly one-quarter have mental health problems. Half of those—more than thirteen thousand people—were diagnosed with post-traumatic stress disorder.[3] The Iraq War is also unusual in that one in every ten U.S. soldiers in Iraq is female,[4] meaning that female soldiers are being exposed to traumatic situations and developing PTSD at levels never seen before.

Many men and women who reenter (or to use the military term, "reintegrate") home life after having been in this intense environment exhibit distinct symptoms. They maintain a combat sensibility long after leaving the battlefield. They are always on edge, mentally on alert, and keenly attuned to the smallest change in their physical setting. To be otherwise would risk death in a war zone, but in civilian life such attitudes can lead to unnecessary stress for the veteran, as well as disturbing his or her family, friends, and associates. While many soldiers "wind down" from a combat-ready mentality in a reasonable amount of time, others are incapable of doing so. They may need weeks or months to regain the emotional equilibrium civilians call "normalcy." Some never return to "normal" and become isolated and alienated from the society in which they live.

Getting Treatment

During previous wars when PTSD was not well understood by society and the medical community, it could be difficult for veterans to get treatment. This has changed since the official diagnosis of PTSD was developed in the 1980s. Treatment is now more common. The military and the Department of Veterans Affairs (VA) have attempted to detect signs of PTSD early and provide treatment. In 2006 the Department of Defense issued new mental health guidelines that expand screening for troops about to be deployed and set limits on when soldiers with psychiatric problems can be kept in combat.[5] Teams of counselors, chaplains, and other mental health professionals were sent into the field to work with soldiers serving in Iraq. They use questionnaires and group therapy sessions to ascertain the mental readiness of the soldiers in their command. There are questions about how effective the military can really be in spotting and dealing with signs of PTSD among soldiers in the field, however. The military sincerely desires to keep its soldiers healthy, but the nature of the military's mission in Iraq requires that the soldiers there be put into dangerous situations. Furthermore, given the need to keep as many soldiers in the field as possible, there is pressure to keep even those who may be developing PTSD or other mental illnesses serving.

The soldiers themselves also present challenges to treating PTSD. In previous wars and in previous generations, soldiers were expected to "get over" the experience of being in combat. It was considered unmanly, even shameful, to dwell on the bad or negative aspects of war. Many veterans kept their wartime experiences private, or only shared them with fellow soldiers. While today's soldiers and veterans are more open about their experiences, many remain reluctant to admit to suffering from PTSD. There is still a real stigma among soldiers about admitting to being psychologically wounded by the experiences of war.

Soldiers depend on each other to be strong. They work together in situations where their lives depend on each other. When a soldier feels his friends and fellow soldiers are counting on him or her, that soldier may feel that seeking treatment for PTSD or other disorders is letting them down. Given the military emphasis on strength, soldiers may also fear being ridiculed or shamed by their fellow soldiers if they admit to the "weakness" of PTSD, not to mention the difficulty they may have on a personal level accepting that they are in need of help. On top of all this is the fear that seeking help for psychological problems might jeopardize future promotions, or result in being forced out of active duty. "There's a strange pressure on these soldiers not to have any problems with what they are doing. It's that old idea that a real man and a true warrior will stand strong," said Washington State psychologist Michael Phillips, a trauma specialist who works with vets. Most soldiers, said Phillips, first try to handle problems by themselves. It's not until they see a pattern, or others point it out, that they may finally seek help, if they do so even then.[6] Instead of professional treatment, they may seek relief from PTSD in drugs, alcohol, or suicide.

Reforming the System

Soldiers with serious health problems that prevent them from serving in the field are cared for by the military. If they are discharged from the military—either because their injuries are too severe for them to serve or for other reasons—they are cared for by the U.S. Department of Veterans Affairs, also known as the Veterans Administration or the VA. The VA is the main provider of medical treatment for veterans and the single largest health-care provider in the United States. The military health-care system and that of the VA face the enormous burden of dealing with the physical and mental problems of soldiers returning from Iraq, as well as the medical care of veterans of America's earlier wars. As recent reports attest, soldiers wounded in Iraq receive some of the best traumatic injury care in existence. It is one of the reasons why soldiers are surviving injuries that would have killed them under earlier circumstances. Care for the psychologically wounded lags far behind physical care, however. While the VA's spending on mental health care has increased, that increase is not keeping step with demand, says one recent newspaper report.[7] Meanwhile, on military bases there are shortages of psychologists and psychiatrists and long waits for appointments. Relatively few military mental health professionals have been trained in recommended post-traumatic stress disorder treatments. And when evidence points to the disorder, only 22 percent of soldiers get referrals, a report by the Government Accountability Office found in 2006.[8]

The bureaucracy of the military and the VA is another stumbling block in accessing treatment for PTSD. Each soldier returning from combat diagnosed with PTSD has to file an application for treatment and then wait for the application to be processed. Faced with hundreds of thousands of applications for antidepressants, psychotherapy, hospitalization, and referral to a treatment center, the VA has developed a large backlog. In the meantime, needy soldiers go without care. In the spring of 2007 an independent panel assessed the rundown condition of facilities at the military's Walter Reed Army Medical Center and the red tape wounded Iraq War veterans must go through to access care. The panel's report called the current system for assessing soldiers' disabilities "extremely cumbersome, inconsistent, and confusing," saying it must be "completely overhauled." It called for the creation of a "center of excellence" on treatment, training, and research on two conditions suffered by thousands of troops in Iraq: traumatic brain injury and post-traumatic stress disorder.[9]

Change does not come easy to any bureaucracy and the VA is no different in this regard. Like all bureaucracies, it is reluctant to alter procedures that have been in place for decades. Most observers say the Veterans Administration provides outstanding care for the nation's twenty-four million vets but is overwhelmed by the needs of returning Iraq War soldiers, many of whom will need long-term care. That care is supposed to take place in a seamless fashion once a veteran is transferred from a VA hospital to the benefits system. The transition is where the VA is failing, families of vets complain. They describe mountains of paperwork and forms to complete and lack of personnel to help. Many vets, especially those with debilitating injuries or mental illness, cannot manage all the paperwork themselves and fall through the cracks.

Kinds of Treatment

Researchers are working on finding new drug therapies and new forms of psychological counseling for the treatment of PTSD. Cognitive-behavioral therapy treats PTSD by teaching the patient to change the way they think about their trauma. Therapists help patients to understand that they are not to blame for the trauma that occurred, that the trauma will not happen again, and that they are safe. Antidepressant medications can also be helpful in reducing the symptoms of PTSD.

Another method being used to treat the symptoms of PTSD is exposure therapy. This mode of therapy involves exposing the patient to the traumatic event that triggered his PTSD, but doing so in a safe environment that will allow the patient to learn that the trauma is in the past. The goal is to reduce the emotional response linked with the events. This exposure can take the form of simply talking about the traumatic event with therapists. Advanced technology can take prolonged exposure therapy further. One army medical center tested virtual reality technology in which a soldier wears a helmet through which he or she views a 360-degree image of a scenario such as a foot patrol in a city neighborhood or a convoy making its way across a desert. The scenarios can be changed to fit the soldier's unique experience.[10]

Some psychologists disagree with exposure therapy, however. They say that it is difficult to correctly diagnose PTSD and that many individuals so diagnosed are also depressed and anxious. In such cases, exposure to the trauma might be counterproductive since the trauma might be worsened by underlying depression and anxiety. These skeptics doubt whether one trauma, such as exposure to war, could be at the root of so much mental illness.

Education, Funding, and Expanding Treatment

Many psychologists are optimistic about successfully treating PTSD. They point to drug therapies and counseling therapies as proven methods. They also believe that the public is more educated about the illness, its causes, and its consequences and is therefore able to extend help when it is needed. Communities are also organizing support groups for veterans and their families.

Nevertheless, addressing the needs of veterans with PTSD is a daunting task. Most veterans returning from Iraq are very young and many may require years of treatment. In the worst cases, some may develop chronic mental illness. Advocates for veterans argue that government spending on treating the mental and physical health problems of war veterans, currently budgeted in the hundreds of billions of dollars, must increase if an entire generation is to regain health and productivity.

Policy makers, veterans, and veterans' families are demanding more services and better care. They are leading the call for changes and improvements in the system. These involve streamlining the paperwork required for accessing care, establishing specialized services for vets with PTSD in smaller cities and rural areas, and extending the hours of clinics to coincide with the soldiers' work schedules. Many more vet centers, storefront outreach and counseling centers built to care for Vietnam veterans, will have to be built and staffed to cater to the needs of the Iraq veterans. And the VA will have to include treatment for mental health and substance abuse in all of its facilities.

The challenges faced by veterans with PTSD are unique in many ways, but they also reflect the overall state of mental health care in the United States. Mental illnesses of all types carries with it a stigma that, like PTSD, can discourage those who are suffering from seeking treatment. For those who do want treatment, it can be difficult to get. The mentally ill, be they veterans with PTSD or civilians with other disorders, are not always capable of dealing with the complicated network of health-care professionals, government agencies, and insurance companies that make up the mental health-care system. And, finding qualified and affordable providers can be difficult for veterans and civilians alike.

Notes

1. Raney Aronson, "Soldiers Heart," PBS, March 1, 2005, www.pbs.org/wgbh/pages/frontline/shows/heart/Frontline.
2. Mark Greer, "A New Kind of War. With Thousands of Returning Troops Who May Need Help Battling Trauma, Civilian and Military Psychologists Alike Are Finding New Ways to Help," APA Online, www.apa.org/monitor/apr05/war.html.
3. Jeremy Manier and Judith Graham, "Veterans Fight the War Within," *Chicago Tribune*, March 12, 2007, www.tilrc.org/docs/0307within.htm.
4. Sara Corbett, "The Women's War," *New York Times Magazine*, March 19, 2007.
5. Matthew Kauffman and Lisa Chedekel, "More Resources Needed, Panel Is Told; Witnesses: Iraq War Putting Strain on Troops and System for Providing Mental Health Care," *Hartford Courant*, December 21, 2006.
6. M.L. Lyke, "The Unseen Cost of War: American Minds Soldiers Can Sustain Psychological Wounds for a Lifetime," *Seattle Post-Intelligencer*, August 27, 2004, http://seattlepi.nwsource.com/local/188143_ptsd27.html.
7. Charles M. Sennot, "Straining to Keep a Promise," *Boston Globe*, March 11, 2007.
8. Manier and Graham, *Chicago Tribune*, March 12, 2007.
9. Scott Shane, "Panel on Walter Reed Woes Issues Strong Rebuke," *New York Times*, April 12, 2007, www.nytimes.com/2007/04/12/washington/12medical.html?hp.
10. Rachel Young, "New Virtual PTSD Treatment," Military.com, March 24, 2007, http://military.com/features.

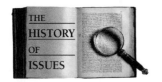

CHAPTER 1

Mental Health in Early American History

Chapter Preface

Mental illness was poorly understood during the earliest period of American history. Colonists in the seventeenth century were likely to explain mental illnesses in religious or mystical terms. With no truly effective treatments available, society's main concern was that the mentally ill be looked after and kept from harming themselves or others. Called the "distracted" or "lunatick," the mentally ill of colonial America were primarily kept at home where their families cared for them. They were also a drag on the economic life of their settlement because they could not generally work and had to be clothed, housed, and fed by someone else. These factors colored the actions taken by the colonies in dealing with the mad.

This is not to say that society as a whole felt no responsibility toward the mentally ill. If an insane person lost his or her family, then, generally speaking, their community would provide for him or her. If a family was too poor or unable to take care of their insane family member, then the community would often give aid in the form of a subsidy. These forms of welfare were highly informal, however, and varied according to each situation.

In time the colonies saw the need to take formal action for their insane citizens so that no one person or group would be required to bear the burden alone. The growth of the colonies and the increasing number of mentally ill persons saw colonial officials instituting codes that spelled out how the insane should be taken care of. In 1641 the Massachusetts Bay Colony led the way when it adopted a code authorizing "allowances" and "dispensations" for the insane. Massachusetts soon made all insane persons without families the legal responsibility of the community.

Other colonies instituted their own codes or copied Massachusetts' model of providing for the care of the insane, the poor, the orphaned, or the needy newcomer. In this respect the American colonies followed precedents established in the mother country. England had a system of poor laws since medieval times and built workhouses and poorhouses to shelter both the poor and the dependent insane. The American colonies followed suit and built the first almshouse in Boston in 1662. Other cities soon followed, but no provisions were made for separating the insane from the poor.

Sometimes the behavior of the mentally ill person caused town officials or settlements to take drastic measures. These included banishing mentally ill nonresidents from the community and forcing them to return to their hometowns. Violent individuals were sometimes incarcerated in small houses in the community to keep them from wandering the countryside or harassing their fellow citizens. These places of confinement were usually built at the community's expense. Local officials were given a great deal of latitude in dealing with the insane, but their actions usually combined the practical needs of their town or city with a sense of moral obligation. There were exceptions, however. The fact that the mentally ill were primarily cared for by their family members or local governments allowed for a wide variation in the quality of care they received.

In the eighteenth and nineteenth centuries new ideas began to change how American society thought about the mentally ill. The goal of eighteenth-century physicians such as Dr. Benjamin Rush was to use science to restore the mentally ill to reason instead of simply confining them as societal nuisances. "Mental illness must be freed from moral stigma, and be treated with medicine rather than moralizing," stated Rush in one of his treatises on mental illness. Hospitals where the mentally ill could be given special treatment began to develop. This shift was given added force by social reformers, who argued that the mentally ill should be protected by state and federal governments and not left to the inconsistent, and in some cases neglectful, care of families and communities. This chapter traces the development of early America's attitudes toward mental health from that of a mostly private concern to the beginnings of a centralized mental health-care system.

Mental Disease in the Colonial Period: An Economic and Social Problem

Gerald N. Grob

According to historian Gerald N. Grob, author of the following selection, there were no government policies regarding the care of the mentally ill during America's colonial period. This situation arose due to the small numbers of people living in the colonies and from eighteenth-century attitudes about the role of society with regard to the mentally ill and other dependent persons. As Grob states, colonial families generally took on the responsibility of caring for a mentally ill member, but communities also passed codes and laws for the maintenance of such individuals. In this respect they followed precedents established under English law.

In the language of the 1600s and 1700s, "care" constituted not medical treatment but economic upkeep and, if required, separation of dangerous persons from the rest of the population. And persons other than the mentally ill could be forced to leave a community if local leaders judged that person to be a potential drain on the town's ability to support him or her. Thus, economics was of great importance to colonists in dealing with the mentally ill.

Gerald N. Grob is a professor of history at Rutgers, the State University of New Jersey. He is also the author of From Asylum to Community: Mental Health Policy in Modern America *and* Mental Institutions in America: Social Policy to 1875.

In modern America the mentally ill are highly visible and therefore of public concern. In the seventeenth and eighteenth centuries, by contrast, mentally ill—or, to use the terminology of that age, "distracted" or "lunatick"—persons aroused far less interest. Society was predominantly rural and agricultural, and communities were small and scattered. Mental illnesses were perceived to be an individual rather than a societal problem, to be handled by the family of the disordered person and not by the state. The very concept of social policy—the conscious creation of public policies and institutions to deal with dependency and distress—was virtually unknown.

The absence of systematic policies did not imply that insanity was of no significance. On the contrary, the presence of mentally ill persons was of serious concern to both families and neighbors. The behavior of "distracted" persons might prove a threat to their own safety or that of others, and the inability to work meant that others would have to assume responsibility for their survival. Nevertheless, the proportionately small number of "distracted" persons did not warrant the creation of special facilities. Nor had insanity come under medical jurisdiction; concepts of insanity in that period were fluid and largely arose from cultural, popular, and intellectual sources. Mentally disordered persons, therefore, were cared for on an ad hoc and informal basis either by the family or community. Insanity was an intensely human problem, and families and neighbors made whatever adjustments they deemed logical and necessary to mitigate its consequences to themselves and the community.

Before the American Revolution mental illnesses posed social and economic rather than medical problems. The care of the insane remained a family responsibility; so long as its members could provide the basic necessities of life for afflicted relatives, no other arrangements were required. Yet in many instances the effects of the illness spilled outside the family and into the community. Sometimes the behavior of "lunatics" or "distracted persons" threatened the safety and security of others. James Otis, Jr., an important eighteenth-century Massachusetts politician, went berserk and began "madly firing the guns outside of his window." For the remainder of his life he alternated between lucidity and bizarre behavior. Sometimes afflicted individuals were unable to work and earn enough for sustenance. In other cases the absence of a family required the community to make some provision for care or for guardianship. When one "distracted" person wandered into a Massachusetts town "in most distressed circumstances in most severe weather," local officials insisted that "humanity required [that] care should be taken to prevent her from perishing." She was placed with a local family and provided with the basic necessities of life at public expense while an effort was begun to discover her original place of residence.

Throughout the seventeenth and eighteenth centuries most cases involving the insane arose out of this inability to support themselves. Illnesses, particularly those that were protracted, created unemployment, which in turn had disastrous impact upon the individual as well as the immediate family. If either the husband or wife was affected, the remainder of the family, including dependent children, faced dire economic consequences. Under such circumstances the community was required to assist the insane person and his or her family.

Early colonial laws were based on the English principle that society had a corporate responsibility for the poor and dependent. As in England, most colonies required local communities to make provision for various classes of dependent persons. Since illness and dependency were intimately related, the care of the mentally ill fell under the jurisdiction of the local community. Various codes and laws enacted in Massachusetts, for example, touched upon the care of the insane in one form or another. The first legal code, adopted in 1641, contained several references to "distracted" persons and idiots. One section authorized a "generall Court" to validate the transfer of property made by such persons. Another provision stipulated that "Children, Idiots, Distracted persons, and all that are strangers, or new commers to our plantation, shall have such allowances and dispensations in any Cause whether Criminall or other as religion and reason require." By 1676 the legislature, noting the rise in the number of "distracted persons" and the resulting behavioral problems, ordered town selectmen to care for such persons in order that "they doe not Damnify others." Another statute in 1694 made all insane persons without families the legal responsibility of the community. Its officials were enjoined "to take effectual care and make necessary provision for the relief, support and safety of such impotent or distracted person." If the individual was destitute, the town was required to assume financial responsibility. Other colonies, including Connecticut, New York, Rhode Island, and Vermont followed suit and often copied Bay Colony statutes outright. Even Virginia, which had laws dealing only with the property and status of the insane, cared for them under a poor law system modeled after that of England.

Virtually none of this legislation referred to the medical treatment of the insane; the emphasis was strictly upon the social and economic consequences of mental disorders. This omission was not an oversight. To the limited extent that contemporary medical literature even discussed insanity, the concern was focused largely on the nature rather than treatment of mental disorders. Indeed, specific therapies were rarely mentioned before 1800. The frequent use of bleeding and purging reflected the influence of the Galenic [named after Galen, the ancient Greek physician] humoral tradition. Disease, according to this tradition, was general rather than specific; it followed an excess in the production of any one of the four humors (blood, yellow bile, black bile, and phlegm). The physiological imbalances that resulted were treated by general nonspecific therapies, of which bleeding and purging were the most common. The distinction between mental and physical diseases, therefore, was tenuous at best. The relatively small numbers of trained physicians militated against medicalization as well. Sick individuals were often treated by ministers and women rather than doctors.

Although insanity was not yet defined exclusively in secular and medical terms, explanations about its origins or manifestations abounded. Most individuals who migrated to the New World brought with them the beliefs, traditions, and practices common in England as well as on the continent. Madness in early modern England was a term that conjured up supernatural, religious, astrological, scientific, and medical elements. The boundaries between magic, religion, medicine, and science were virtually nonexistent, and those who wrote about madness could integrate themes and explanations from all to explain mysterious phenomena.

The life of Richard Napier, an early seventeenth-century astrological physician, is illustrative. Napier treated five to fifteen patients per day between 1597 and 1634. During his career thousands of patients consulted him, of whom more than two thousand were either mad or deeply troubled. Like others of his generation, Napier believed that mental disorders could flow from both natural and supernatural sources. Stress, for example, could lead to either physical or mental disturbances. But mental disorders could also follow from the intervention of God as well as the Devil. Napier employed medicaments, psychology, environmental manipulation, and astrology in his armamentarium. He also exorcised those patients he believed to be possessed. When Edmund Francklin was brought before him, Napier ended with the following incantation:

Behold, I God's most unworthy minister and servant, I do charge and command thee, thou cruel beast, with all thy associates and all other malignant spirits in case that any of you have your being in the body of this creature, Mr. E. Fr[ancklin], and have distempered his brain with melancholy and have also deprived his body and limbs of their natural see. I charge and command you speedily to depart from this creature and servant of God, Mr. E. F[rankling], regenerated by the laver of the holy baptism and redeemed by the precious blood of our Lord Jesus Christ, I charge you to depart from him and every part of his body really, personally. . . .

The colonists who settled America brought with them English traditions and practices, including a poor law system that mandated local responsibility for distressed persons. Yet local responsibility had a quite different meaning in America, which lacked large urban areas and complex institutional arrangements characteristic of the mother country. Even outside London—by far the largest metropolitan area in England—population was sufficiently dense as to permit the creation of workhouses and poorhouses (which often held mad persons). London had an elaborate institutional network to care for the mentally ill, including the famous Bethlehem Hospital (often referred to as Bedlam), which held large numbers of dependent insane persons. In America, by contrast, population was widely dispersed. As late as 1790 there were only six areas with more than 8,000 residents; these held only 3.35 percent of the total population. Only two (New York and Philadelphia) had more than 25,000 residents, and none had more than 50,000. Such diffuse populations could not support large institutions to care for the insane. Confinement was the exception rather than the rule.

Unless they threatened public safety, people who were mad resided in the community. Those able to work were often afforded the opportunity to do so. Joseph Moody, a Harvard graduate and minister to a Maine church, wore a handkerchief over his face because of his feelings of unworthiness. During the services he turned his back on the audience for the same reason. His congregation accepted his bizarre ministry for three years, and even after he was removed from his pulpit and preached occasionally, his behavior was unchanged. Similarly, James Otis, Jr., occupied a series of public offices and maintained a law practice even though his obviously irrational behavior placed him beyond the bounds of sanity. Indeed, individuals who could manage their jobs or who recovered from episodes of madness were quickly absorbed into the community even though insanity was by no means free of stigma. Daniel Kirtland, a Yale graduate, lost his ministerial position after becoming insane. Upon his subsequent recovery, he received a comparable appointment from another Connecticut church. . . .

But these tolerant attitudes had limits. When the behavior of insane persons appeared to threaten public safety, more stringent actions followed. Seventeenth- and eighteenth-century legislation often contained clauses empowering local officials to limit the freedom of "distracted persons" who menaced other residents. A Virginia court in 1689 took notice of John Stock, an individual "whoe keepes running about the neighborhood day and night in a sad Distracted Condition to the great Disturbance of the people." To prevent "his doeing any further Mischiefe," the court ordered the sheriff to place Stock "in some close Roome, where hee shall not bee suffered to go abroad untill hee bee in a better condition to Governe himselfe." Fear and benevolence were inextricably intertwined. When a colonial soldier who killed his mother was acquitted by reason of insanity, the court ordered him confined for life to a "small place" erected by his father in his home, but at public expense.

Other communities reacted in a negative manner when confronted with the responsibility of providing for nonresident dependent persons. Such concerns gave rise to the legally sanctioned practice of "warning out"—a practice based on the proposition that towns had the right to exclude strangers. Legal residency during the colonial period was not an inherent right, but rather a privilege granted by existing residents. The distrust of strangers reflected both the relative absence of formal mechanisms of control to deal with behavior that might menace public order and a desire to absolve towns of any financial liability for the support of ill or unemployed strangers. Hence it was not uncommon for local officials to force the return of insane persons to the community in which they were legal residents. As residents of the largest town in New England, Bostonians sometimes found nonresident insane persons in their community. Officials frequently attempted to return such individuals to the town from which they originally came. When sending Edward Eveleth to Ipswich, the Boston selectmen noted that he was "disposed to wander" and requested Ipswich officials to "take care to prevent his returning to us, which if he should will occasion a charge to your Town." The overwhelming majority of individuals "warned out," however, were not insane, suggesting that fiscal concerns rather than fear of insanity shaped this practice. Efforts to avoid or to shift welfare costs became a tradition that was to play a major role in shaping public policy toward mental illnesses during the nineteenth and twentieth centuries.

To most colonial Americans insanity was of concern because of its economic ramifications and potential threat to public safety. Medical considerations played virtually no role in shaping practices and customs. Given prevailing standards of living, available resources, and the absence of institutions, there is every reason to believe that the fate of the insane was not appreciably different from that of other dependent groups. Like widows, orphans, handicapped, aged, and sick persons, insane individuals required public assistance. Although always present, fiscal concerns were softened by long-standing ethical and moral values that assigned an unyielding obligation to assist those unable to survive independently.

Early American Speculations About the "Distracted"

Mary Ann Jimenez

*In her study of insanity in colonial New England, social histo-
rian Mary Ann Jimenez examines early American attitudes toward mental illness. In the following selection from her 1987
monograph on the subject, Jimenez describes the speculations of
the Puritan minister Cotton Mather (1663–1728), the most in-
fluential religious thinker, preacher, and writer in the early colonial period. As Jimenez states, Mather saw a supernatural ele-
ment in mental illness, an attitude he shared with his
contemporaries in the Massachusetts Bay Colony. As a leading
intellect in his community, Mather used the pulpit and the pen
to explain insanity to his congregation as yet another example of
God's limitless and mysterious intervention in human affairs. By
doing so he was in strict keeping with Calvinist theology—which
saw the hand of Divine Providence in all things—by seeing in
mental illness a sign of God's punishment for some moral lapse
or as a test of an individual's resolve. Jimenez also points out
that Mather and his fellow Puritans distinguished between the
melancholia or ravings of the distracted from the behavior of
those possessed by a demon. The insane or "distracted" persons
were to be pitied and not punished as possessed "witches" were
in the infamous Salem witch trials.*

Cotton Mather, the great Puritan divine, was perhaps the
most literate and certainly the most famous observer of
madness in colonial Massachusetts. His speculations about its
nature and causes suggest the complexity of the colonial effort
to understand insanity, in which religious, biological, and

Mary Ann Jimenez, *Changing Faces of Madness: Early American Attitudes and Treatment
of the Insane*, Hanover, NH: Brandeis University Press, University Press of New England,
1987, pp. 12–17. Copyright © 1987 by Trustees of Brandeis University. All rights reserved. Reprinted by permission.

moral explanations were woven into a unified model of madness in which God, devil, and human actors all played various roles.

A Struggle with Satan

Mather's earliest writings about madness emphasized the satanic connection, as in a sermon where he suggested that "there is an unaccountable and unexpressable interest of Satan often times in the Distemper of madness." He rather poetically described how this "interest of Satan" works: "It is often some Devil, which takes advantage of the Poisonous Fires which madness is inflamed with, to carry on the hideous Hurly Burly's that are in the minds of the distempered." How does Satan work through the human body? Mather thought that some men "afford a bed wherein busy and bloody devils have a sort of lodging provided for them." The "bed" is a "mass of blood . . . disordered with some fiery acid," and "juices, ferments and vapours." Alternatively, something may be awry with the humors, which "yield the steams when Satan does insinuate himself until he has gained a sort of possession in them, or at least an opportunity to shoot into the mind as many fiery darts as may cause sad life to them." Of course, Satan was implicated in many untoward occurrences in colonial Massachusetts, most notably witchcraft, but he was also thought to have the power to drive or tempt a person into madness. The responsibility to resist the importuning of the devil rested with those so beset; however, the failure to win the struggle was not necessarily a cause for shame.

William Thompson, a melancholy minister in late seventeenth century Massachusetts, became so debilitated by his mental state that he had to resign his ministry. Mather wrote of him sympathetically in *Magnalia Christi Americana* in 1702, recalling that Satan became "irritated by the evangelic labours of this holy man" and "obtained the liberty to throw him into a Balneum Diaboli." Mather assured his readers that Satan had obtained this "liberty" from God, who finally saved Thompson from his madness, thanks to the prayers of his congregation. While Mather's need to find a moral lesson in Thompson's story has him restored to reason after his congregation's prayers, other accounts have him going to his grave insane.

Resisting the devil's assault on one's sanity was a very strenuous task. In a collection of poems written after his death by Thompson's family and friends, the minister is described as courageously trying to thwart the devil's efforts, as he "vexed his mind with diabolical assaults and horrid, hellish darts." These devilish attacks left Thompson resembling "the lively portrature of Death / A walking tomb, a living sepulcher / In which black melancholy did inter." Although the devil was the primary actor in the onset of Thompson's madness, the poet was careful to acknowledge the ultimate authority of God in allowing the devil to tempt him, for "he hath let the devil loose / me strongly to oppose." While Mather's account of Thompson's suffering leaves the reader with a strong impression of the latter's innocence, in these poems the suggestion appears that Thompson "swerved from the duties of his calling" and so brought on Satan's assaults himself. Here the moral implications of madness are summoned; its appearance could signal some earlier flaw that had given the devil a foothold, just as Mather, on another occasion, suggested that some men offer Satan an easy "bed." Madness, like anything calamitous that might befall the colonist, was a rich source of moral instruction.

Distraction versus Possession

In 1719 Mather pointed out another way in which the devil might be responsible for madness, when he began fretting over his third wife's behavior, which he described as consisting of "furious and froward pangs." He worried whether they were the result of a "distraction or a possession." *Distraction* was the most common name for ordinary madness in colonial Massachusetts, while *possession* suggested a more serious form and implied a direct takeover of an individual's will by Satan. During one "prodigious return of her pangs upon her," Mather's wife Lydia scolded her husband with a "thousand unrepeateable invectives" and "got into a horrid rage," causing him to judge her behavior "Little short of a Proper Satanical Possession."

Possession by the devil might be suggested by the more extreme forms of madness, but such behavior could also summon the specter of witchcraft, a distinct form of Satanic intervention in human affairs. Colonists usually made a distinction between possession and bewitchment, since the latter meant, for one thing, the necessity of finding a witch to prosecute. Mather was probably not worried that his wife was bewitched. He had, after all, witnessed several cases of bewitchment in the course of his ministry and knew that there were "distinct and formal fits of witchcraft" that accompanied true bewitchment. Colonists drew a very clear line between madness, which might or might not be caused by possession, and bewitchment, as evidenced by the efforts of witnesses in cases of suspected bewitchment to rule out madness. The behavior of the bewitched was far more dramatic than that of the merely distracted; in fact, there was an expectation that something "preternatural" should be performed by one who was truly bewitched. Being under the spell of a witch was clearly not the same as being distracted; one dissenter from the Salem witchcraft trials argued that the Salem girls were not bewitched but were merely "poor distracted children," or perhaps "a parcel of possessed, distracted or lying wenches." As Mather knew well, the colonists did not view any part of the witchcraft drama as a sign of anyone's insanity, whether witch or bewitched.

Cotton Mather may not have known how to account for his wife's behavior, but if he *had* really believed that the devil was responsible for her outbursts, he might have been less inclined to blame her. In the case of a minister of Mather's acquaintance whom Satan drove mad, Mather was exceedingly sympathetic. In *Magnalia Christi Americana*, Mather recounted the story of John Warham, a pious man whom Satan "threw into the deadly pangs of melancholy," and who suffered "terrible temptations and buffetings," which were relieved only at his death. Mather was concerned about a growing number of "pious" New Englanders who "have contracted these melancholy indispositions which have unhinged them from all service or comfort." Explaining the madness of apparently good people was occasion for calling upon the "unsearchable judgements of God," who allowed the devil to drive such persons mad. The melancholy forms of madness may have been viewed in a more sympathetic light than were the raving kinds. In another sermon written in 1717, Mather argues that melancholy madness, the kind suffered by those with "troubled minds," was likely to be a test by God of the patience and resolve of an otherwise holy person.

Using Madness to Teach a Moral Lesson

Mather found insanity somewhat easier to explain when the afflicted person clearly had been guilty of some moral transgression. In *Magnalia* he pointed out the case, "which many hundreds among us know to be true," of a layman who, upon being asked to preach a sermon for an absent minister, took the opportunity to attack the exclusive right of the clergy to preach. Mather warned the reader that this sin of pride was immediately punished, when "God smote him with a horrible madness; he was taken ravingly distracted: the people were forced with violent hands to carry him home." He lived the rest of his life in total madness, according to the minister's account. Here the raving madness of an obvious sinner was easily translated into a moral lesson.

Sin was not the cause only of insanity in Mather's cosmology, but of all human suffering. It was, he argued in "Insanibilia," the cause of "all the grievous things" that come from God. This view of sin as an all-purpose agent of human misery was shared by Mather's contemporaries in the early eighteenth century, yet their emphasis on human responsibility for suffering did not eliminate the role of Satan, for he still had a "hand in All grievous Things which darken the world."

Mather combined supernatural actors, personal sin, and human biology to explain madness in the early eighteenth century. His causal scheme was flexible; the distraction of the saint was understood as another of God's tests of his followers, while the sinner could be blamed for bringing on his own insensibility by invoking God's punishment. The devil could be summoned in either case: as a way of blaming those who did not resist his blandishments, or as the overpowering force that swept aside the rationality of an unwilling victim.

Mather was writing as a Puritan minister, one who would be eager to explain insanity in religious terms. His views are important not only because of his eminence in colonial Massachusetts, but also because they were probably shared by most of his contemporaries. The Massachusetts Bay colonists were very likely to believe in the reality of the supernatural order invoked by Mather, and they had much evidence of the direct power of God and the devil in their lives. What we would call superstitious beliefs in witchcraft, in signs and portents, were widespread in the colony in this period, in urban as well as in rural areas. These beliefs were part of a complex framework of causality in which all happenings, including those with natural causes, such as earthquakes and storms, were seen in a supernatural light. The colonists believed that God's hand was in all events, and they were particularly eager to point to this in the case of anything untoward.

Mather's explanations of madness were fashioned out of a traditional model that included a powerful demonology, a strong sense of sin, and an acceptance of God's ultimate power. His speculations about madness remind us that the division between secular and religious reality that characterizes modern thinking was not so important in colonial thinking. Calvinism [the Christianity of the Puritans] provided a symbolic structure that lent supernatural meaning to all human activities. This ability to explain the everyday aspects of reality in supernatural terms was especially important when no other clear explanation existed. The rational basis of Puritanism did not completely eliminate the belief in the basic inscrutability of God, which allowed every event, no matter how untoward, to be absorbed into the predominant symbolic order of Calvinist theology. The notion of Providence was an all-encompassing concept that explained God's mysterious intervention into human affairs. Puritans believed that God's Providence was not passive but consisted in the direct operation of His will in the natural order. God's inscrutability as well as His glory was therefore magnified by the appearance of the unusual. In the last analysis, madness was another way this lesson could be learned more profoundly.

The Medical Treatment of Mental Illness: The Work of Benjamin Rush

Robert Whitaker

By the late 1700s doctors in America began to follow the techniques of their European counterparts in treating mental illness as a disease. This meant forming hypotheses as to the biological causes of mental illness and inventing therapies for the relief of suffering. Those therapies included such measures as bloodletting, purges, and hydrotherapy, all of which were regarded as helpful to the patient. This evolution in the treatment of the mentally ill is the subject of the following article by journalist and author Robert Whitaker. In it he traces the beginnings of modern psychiatry with a special focus on the career of physician Benjamin Rush (1745–1813) of Pennsylvania Hospital and author of Medical Inquiries and Observations upon Diseases of the Mind, *the first American textbook of psychiatry. As Whitaker points out, Rush inhabited two worlds: As a Quaker and social reformer, he believed that the mentally ill should be treated with kindness and compassion. He was also a man of science who was eager to introduce the latest European practices in his American hospital. These practices involved physically weakening the mentally ill in order to make them docile and inspiring fear and dread on the part of the ill. Such hazardous practices—regarded as humane in the eighteenth century—would dominate the treatment of the mentally ill for years to come.*

Robert Whitaker is a journalist who writes about medicine and science. He is also the author of The Mapmaker's Wife.

A visitor to the "mad" wards of Pennsylvania Hospital at the turn of the nineteenth century would have found the halls astir with an air of reform. A few years earlier, in 1796 to be exact, the lunatics had been moved from unheated, dingy cells in the basement, where they had often slept on straw and been confined in chains, to a new wing, where their rooms were above ground. Here the winter chill was broken by a coal-fired stove, and occasionally the mad patients could even take a warm bath. Most important of all, they now began to receive regular medical treatments—a regimen of care, physician Benjamin Rush proudly told the Pennsylvania Hospital overseers, that had "lately been discovered to be effectual in treating their disorder."

The introduction of medical treatments had been a long time coming. In 1751, when Quakers and other community leaders in Philadelphia had petitioned the Pennsylvania colonial assembly for funds to build the hospital, the first in the colonies, they had told of medical care that could help restore sanity to the mad mind. "It has been found," wrote Benjamin Franklin, who authored the plea, "by the experience of many Years, that above two Thirds of the Mad People received into Bethlehem Hospital [in England] and there treated properly, have been perfectly cured." English mad-doctors had indeed begun making such claims and had even published books describing their effective treatments. However, while Franklin and his fellow Quakers may have hoped to bring such medicine to the colonies, they also had a second reason for building the hospital. There were, they wrote, too many lunatics "going at large [who] are a Terror to their neighbors, who are daily apprehensive of the Violences they may commit." Society needed to be protected from the insane, and it was this second function—hospital as jail—that had taken precedence when the hospital opened in 1756.

In those early years, the lunatics were kept in gloomy, foul-smelling cells and were ruled over by "keepers" who used their whips freely. Unruly patients, when not being beaten, were regularly "chained to rings of iron, let into the floor or wall of the cell . . . restrained in hand-cuffs or ankle-irons," and bundled into Madd-shirts that "left the patient an impotent bundle of wrath." . . . All of this began to change once Rush arrived at the hospital in 1783.

A Champion of Reform

The lunatics could not have hoped for a more kind-hearted man to be their advocate. Born of Quaker parents, Rush was constantly championing liberal, humanitarian reforms. As a young man, he had been a member of the Continental Congress and a signer of the Declaration of Independence. He'd advocated for the abolition of slavery and prison reform, and he brought this same compassion to his treatment of the mad. At his request, the hospital's governing board built a new wing for the insane patients, which was completed in 1796, and soon many patients were enjoying the comforts of rooms furnished with hair mattresses and feather beds. Those who were well behaved were allowed to stroll about the hospital grounds and engage in activities like sewing, gardening, and cutting straw. Rush also believed that games, music, and friendship could prove helpful, and the hospital even agreed to his request that "a Well qualified Person be employed as a Friend and Companion to the Lunatics." The insane, he explained to hospital attendants, needed to be treated with kindness and respect. "Every thing necessary for their comfort should be provided for them, and every promise made to them should be faithfully and punctually performed."

But such humanitarian care could only go so far. Rush was also a man of science. He'd studied at the University of Edinburgh, the most prestigious medical school in the world at the time. There, he'd been mentored by the great William Cullen, whose *First Lines of the Practice of Physic* was perhaps the leading medical text of the day. The European mad-doctors had developed a diverse array of therapeutics for curing madness, and Rush, eager to make Pennsylvania Hospital a place of modern medicine, employed their methods with great vigor. And this was treatment of an altogether different type. . . .

Taming and Weakening the Ill

[Medical science in Rush's time held that] lunatics needed to be dominated and broken. The primary treatments advocated by English physicians were those that physically weakened the mad—bleeding to the point of fainting and the regular use of powerful purges, emetics, and nausea-inducing agents. All of this could quickly reduce even the strongest maniac to a pitiful, whimpering state. William Cullen, reviewing bleeding practices, noted that some advised cutting into the jugular vein. Purges and emetics, which would make the mad patient violently sick, were to be repeatedly administered over an extended period. John Monro, superintendent of [London's] Bethlehem Asylum, gave one of his patients sixty-one vomit-inducing emetics in six months, including strong doses on eighteen successive nights. Mercury and other chemical agents, meanwhile, were used to induce nausea so fierce that the patient could not hope to have the mental strength to rant and rave. "While nausea lasts," George Man Burrows advised, "hallucinations of long adherence will be suspended, and sometimes be perfectly removed, or perhaps exchanged for others, and the most furious will become tranquil and obedient." It was, he added, "far safer to reduce the patient by nauseating him than by depleting him."

A near-starvation diet was another recommendation for robbing the madman of his strength. The various depleting remedies—bleedings, purgings, emetics, and nausea-inducing agents—were also said to be therapeutic because they inflicted considerable pain, and thus the madman's mind became focused on this sensation rather than on his usual raving thoughts. Blistering was another treatment useful for stirring great bodily pain. Mustard powders could be rubbed on a shaved scalp, and once the blisters formed, a caustic was rubbed into the blisters to further irritate and infect the scalp. "The suffering that attends the formation of these pustules is often indescribable," wrote one physician. The madman's pain could be expected to increase as he rubbed his hands in the caustic and touched his genitals, a pain that would enable the patient to "regain consciousness of his true self, to wake from his supersensual slumber and to stay awake."

All of these physically depleting, painful therapies also had a psychological value: They were feared by the lunatics, and thus the mere threat of their employment could get the lunatics to behave in a better manner. Together with liberal use of restraints and an occasional beating, the mad would learn to cower before their doctors and attendants. "In most cases it has appeared to be necessary to employ a very constant impression of fear; and therefore to inspire them with the awe and dread of some particular persons, especially of those who are to be constantly near them," Cullen wrote. "This awe and dread is therefore, by one means or other, to be acquired; in the first place by their being the authors of all the restraints that may be occasionally proper; but sometimes it may be necessary to acquire it even by stripes and blows. The former, although having the appearance of more severity, are much safer than strokes or blows about the head.". . .

In this era of medical optimism, English physicians—and their counterparts in other European countries—developed an ever more innovative array of therapeutics. Dunking the patient in water became quite popular—a therapy intended both to cool the patient's scalp and to provoke terror. Physicians advised pouring buckets of water on the patient from a great height or placing the patient under a waterfall; they also devised machines and pumps that could pummel the patient with a torrent of water. The painful blasts of water were effective "as a remedy and a punishment," one that made patients "complain of pain as if the lateral lobes of the cerebrum were split asunder." The Bath of Surprise became a staple of many asylums: The lunatic, often while being led blindfolded across a room, would suddenly be dropped through a trap-door into a tub of cold water—the unexpected plunge hopefully inducing such terror that the patient's senses might be dramatically restored. . . .

The most common mechanical device to be employed in European asylums during this period was a swinging chair. Invented by Englishman Joseph Mason Cox, the chair could, in one fell swoop, physically weaken the patient, inflict great pain, and invoke terror—all effects perceived as therapeutic for the mad. The chair, hung from a wooden frame, would be rotated rapidly by an operator to induce in the patient "fatigue, exhaustion, pallor, horripilatio [goose bumps], vertigo, etc.," thereby producing "new associations and trains of thoughts." In the hands of a skilled operator, able to rapidly alter the directional motion of the swing, it could reliably produce nausea, vomiting, and violent convulsions. Patients would also involuntarily urinate and defecate, and plead for the machine to be stopped. The treatment was so powerful, said one nineteenth-century physician, that if the swing didn't make a mad person obedient, nothing would. . . .

Rush's Concept of Mental Illness

It was with those teachings in mind that Rush introduced medical treatments into the regimen of care at Pennsylvania Hospital. Although he was a Quaker, a reformist, and one who could empathize with the unfortunate, he was also an educated man, confident in the powers of science, and that meant embracing the practices advocated in Europe. "My first principles in medicine were derived from Dr. [Hermann] Boerhaave," he wrote, citing as his inspiration the very physician who had dreamed up drowning therapy. Moreover, at the time, he and other leading American doctors were struggling to develop an academic foundation for their profession, with European medicine the model to emulate. Before the American Revolution, fewer than 5 percent of the 3,500 doctors in the country had degrees, and only about 10 percent had any formal training at all. Medicine in colonial America had a well-deserved reputation as a refuge for quacks. But that was changing. In 1765, the first medical school in America had been established at the College of Philadelphia, where Rush was one of the faculty members. In the 1790s, medical societies were formed, and the first periodical medical journal was published. It all led to a proud sense of achievement—American medicine was now a scientific discipline. . . .

Rush's conception of madness reflected the teachings of his European mentors. He believed that madness was caused by "morbid and irregular" actions in the blood vessels of the brain. This abnormal circulation of the blood, he wrote, could be due to any number of physical or psychological causes. An injury to the brain, too much labor, extreme weather, worms, consumption, constipation, masturbation, intense study, and too much imagination could all cause a circulatory imbalance. To fix this circulatory disorder, he advocated the copious bleeding of patients, particularly those with mania. He drew 200 ounces of blood from one patient in less than two months; in another instance, he bled a manic patient forty-seven times, removing nearly four gallons of blood. As much as "four-fifths of the blood in the body" should be drawn away, he said. His bleeding regimen was so extreme that other doctors publicly criticized it as a "murderous dose" and a "dose for a horse," barbs that Rush dismissed as the talk of physicians competing "for business and money."

As he employed other remedies he'd learned from the Europeans, he did so in ways that fit his belief that madness was due to a circulatory disorder. For instance, he argued that blisters should be raised on the ankles rather than the scalp, as this would draw blood away from the overheated head. Caustics could be applied to the back of the neck, the wound kept open for months or even years, as this would induce a "permanent discharge" from the overheated brain. The head could also be directly treated. The scalp could be shaved and cold water and ice dumped on the overheated brain. Purges and emetics could also draw blood away from the inflamed brain to the stomach and other organs. Rush administered all of these treatments confident that they were scientific and worked by helping to normalize blood flow in the brain.

Although Rush constantly preached the need to treat the insane in a kind manner, at times he adopted the language of his English teachers, comparing lunatics to the "tyger, the mad bull, and the enraged dog." Intimidation tactics could be used to control them; patients might even be threatened with death. "Fear," he said, "accompanied with pain and a sense of shame, has sometimes cured this disease." A doctor in Georgia, he recounted, had successfully cured a madman by dropping him into a well, the lunatic nearly drowning before he was taken out. Concluded Rush: "Terror acts powerfully upon the body, through the medium of the mind, and should be employed in the cure of madness.". . .

Rush was particularly proud of the "Tranquilizer Chair" he invented, which he boasted could "assist in curing madness." Once strapped into the chair, lunatics could not move at all—their arms were bound, their wrists immobilized, their feet clamped together—and their sight was blocked by a wooden contraption confining the head. A bucket was placed beneath the seat for defecation, as patients would be restrained for long periods at a time. Rush wrote:

> It binds and confines every part of the body. By keeping the trunk erect, it lessens the impetus of blood toward the brain. By preventing the muscles from acting, it prevents the force and frequency of the pulse, and by the position of the head and feet favors the easy application of cold water or ice to the former and warm water to the latter. Its effects have

been truly delightful to me. It acts as a sedative to the tongue and temper as well as to the blood vessels. In 24, 12, six and in some cases in four hours, the most refractory patients have been composed. I call it a Tranquilizer. . . .

Rush stood at the very pinnacle of American medicine at that time. He was the young country's leading authority on madness, and other American physicians copied his ways. They too would bleed their insane patients and weaken them with purges, emetics, and nausea-inducing drugs. Physicians familiar with his teachings might also use water therapies.

Dorothea Dix Advocates for the Humane Treatment of the Mentally Ill

Dorothea Dix

In 1843 humanitarian and social reformer Dorothea Dix (1802–1887) submitted the following pamphlet to the Massachusetts State legislature. In it she called upon the legislators to take up the cause of the mentally ill who were living in subhuman conditions within the state's jails and poorhouses. Dix, a former schoolteacher, was first exposed to social reform when she visited England in the 1830s. Upon her return to the United States, she launched an investigation into the conditions of the mentally ill in Massachusetts. Dix visited jails and almshouses (or houses for the poor) and noted how the insane were chained, beaten into submission, or neglected. The state responded to her call to action and built asylums for the care of the insane. Dix continued her work on behalf of the mentally ill in other states including New Hampshire, Louisiana, and Pennsylvania. Like her fellow reformers Horace Mann and William Lloyd Garrison, Dix believed that citizens were required to correct abuses within their society and extend aid to the less fortunate.

Gentleman.—I respectfully ask to present this Memorial, believing that the cause, which actuates to and sanctions so unusual a movement, presents no equivocal to claim to public consideration and sympathy. . . .

About two years since leisure afforded opportunity and duty prompted me to visit several prisons and almshouses in the vicinity of this metropolis. I found, near Boston, in the jails and asylums for the poor, a numerous class brought into unsuitable connection with criminals and the general mass of

Dorothea Dix, "Memorial to the Massachusetts Legislature (1843)." http://usinfo.state.gov/usa/infousa/facts/democrac/15.htm.

paupers, I refer to idiots and insane persons, dwelling in circumstances not only adverse to their own physical and moral improvement, but productive of extreme disadvantages to all other persons brought into association with them. I applied myself diligently to trace the causes of these evils, and sought to supply remedies. As one obstacle was surmounted, fresh difficulties appeared. Every new investigation has given depth to the conviction that it is only by decided, prompt, and vigorous legislation the evils to which I refer, and which I shall proceed more fully to illustrate, can be remedied. I shall be obliged to speak with great plainness, and to reveal many things revolting to the taste, and from which my woman's nature shrinks with peculiar sensitiveness. But truth is the highest consideration. I tell what I have seen—painful and shocking as the details often are—that from them you may feel more deeply the imperative obligation which lies upon you to prevent the possibility of a repetition or continuance of such outrages upon humanity. . . .

I come to present the strong claims of suffering humanity. I come to place before the Legislature of Massachusetts the condition of the miserable, the desolate, the outcast. I come as the advocate of helpless, forgotten, insane, and idiotic men and women: of beings sunk to a condition from which the most unconcerned would start with real horror: of beings wretched in our prisons, and more wretched in our almshouses. . . .

I must confine myself to few examples, but am ready to furnish other and more complete details, if required.

If my pictures are displeasing, coarse, and severe, my subjects, it must be recollected, offer no tranquil, refined, or composing features. The condition of human beings, reduced to the extremest states of degradation and misery cannot be exhibited in softened language, or adorn a polished page.

I proceed, gentlemen, briefly to call your attention to the present state of insane persons confined within this Commonwealth, in cages, closets, cellars, stalls, pens! Chained, naked, beaten with rods, and lashed into obedience. . . .

The State Is Accountable

It is the Commonwealth, not its integral parts, that is accountable for most of the abuses which have lately and do still exist. I repeat it, it is defective legislation which perpetuates and multiplies these abuses. In illustration of my subject, I offer the following extracts from my Note-book and Journal:—

Springfield. In the jail, one lunatic woman, furiously mad, a State pauper, improperly situated, both in regard to the prisoners, the keepers, and herself. It is a case of extreme self-forgetfulness and oblivion to all the decencies of life, to describe which would be to repeat only the grossest scenes. She is much worse since leaving Worcester [site of a state hospital founded in 1830]. In the almshouse of the same town is a woman apparently only needing judicious care, and some well-chosen employment, to make it unnecessary to confine her in solitude, in a dreary unfurnished room. Her appeals for employment and companionship are most touching, but the mistress replied she had no time to attend to her. . . .

Lincoln. A woman in a cage. Medford. One idiotic subject chained, and one in a close stall for seventeen years. Pepperell. One often doubly chained, hand and foot; another violent; several peaceable now; Brookfield. One man caged, comfortable. Granville. One often closely confined: now losing the use of his limbs from want of exercise. Charlemont. One man caged. Savoy. One man caged. Lenox. Two in the jail. against whose unfit condition there the jailer protests.

Dedham. The insane disadvantageously placed in the jail. In the almshouse, two females in stalls, situated in the main building; lie in wooden bunks filled with straw; always shut up. One of these subjects is supposed curable. The overseers of the poor have declined giving her a trial at the hospital, as I was informed, on account of expense. . . .

Besides the above, I have seen many who, part of the year, are chained or caged. The use of cages all but universal. Hardly a town but can refer to some not distant period of using them; chains are less common; negligences frequent; wilful abuse less frequent than sufferings proceeding from ignorance, or want of consideration. I encountered during the last three months many poor creatures wandering reckless and unprotected through the country. . . . But I cannot particularize. In traversing the State, I have found hundreds of insane persons in every variety of circumstance and condition, many whose situation could not and need not be improved; a less number, but that very large, whose lives are the saddest pictures of human suffering and degradation.

I give a few illustrations; but description fades before reality.

An Almshouse

Danvers. November. Visited the almshouse. A large building, much out of repair. Understand a new one is in contemplation. Here are from fifty-six to sixty inmates, one idiotic, three insane; one of the latter in close confinement at all times.

Long before reaching the house, wild shouts, snatches of rude songs, imprecations and obscene language, fell upon the ear, proceeding from the occupant of a low building, rather remote from the principal building to which my course was directed. Found the mistress, and was conducted to the place which was called "the home" of the forlorn maniac, a young woman, exhibiting a condition of neglect and misery blotting out the faintest idea of comfort, and outraging every sentiment of decency. She had been, I learnt, "a respectable person, industrious and worthy. Disappointments and trials shook her mind, and, finally, laid prostrate reason and self-control. She became a maniac for life. She had been at Worcester Hospital for a considerable time, and had been returned as incurable." The mistress told me she understood that. "while there, she was comfortable and decent." Alas, what a change was here exhibited! She had passed from one degree of violence to another, in swift progress. There she stood, clinging to or beating upon the bars of her caged apartment, the contracted size of which afforded space only for increasing accumulations of filth, a foul spectacle. There she stood with naked arms and dishevelled hair, the unwashed frame invested with fragments of unclean garments, the air so extremely offensive, though ventilation was afforded on all sides save one, that it was not possible to remain beyond a few moments without retreating for recovery to the outward air. Irritation of body, produced by utter filth and exposure, incited her to the horrid process of tearing off her skin by inches. Her face, neck, and person were thus disfigured to hideousness. She held up a fragment just rent off. To my exclamation of horror, the mistress replied: "Oh, we can't help it. Half the skin is off sometimes. We can do nothing with her; and it makes no difference what she eats, for she consumes her own filth as readily as the food which is brought her."

Men of Massachusetts, I beg, I implore, I demand pity and protection for these of my suffering, outraged sex. Fathers, husbands, brothers, I would supplicate you for this boon; but what do I say? I dishonor you, divest you at once of Christianity and humanity, does this appeal imply distrust. If it comes burdened with a doubt of your righteousness in this legislation, then blot it out; while I declare confidence in your honor, not less than your humanity. Here you will put away the cold, calculating spirit of selfishness and self-seeking; lay off the armor of local strife and political opposition; here and now, for once, forgetful of the earthly and perishable, come up to these halls and consecrate them with one heart and one mind to works of righteousness and just judgment.

A Sacred Cause

Become the benefactors of your race, the just guardians of the solemn rights you hold in trust. Raise up the fallen, succor the desolate, restore the outcast, defend the helpless, and for your eternal and great reward receive the benediction, "Well done, good and faithful servants, become rulers over many things!"

Injustice is also done to the convicts: it is certainly very wrong that they should be doomed day after day and night after night to listen to the ravings of madmen and madwomen. This is a kind of punishment that is not recognized by our statutes, and is what the criminal ought not to be called upon to undergo. The confinement of the criminal and of the insane in the same building is subversive of that good order and discipline which should be observed in every well-regulated prison. I do most sincerely hope that more permanent provision will be made for the pauper insane by the State, either to restore Worcester Insane Asylum to what it was originally designed to be or else make some just appropriation for the benefit of this very unfortunate class of our "fellow-beings."

Gentlemen, I commit to you this sacred cause. Your action upon this subject will affect the present and future condition of hundreds and of thousands. In this legislation, as in all things, may you exercise that "wisdom which is the breath of the power of God." Respectfully Submitted, D. L. Dix

A President Rejects a Reformer's Plea

Franklin Pierce

Social reformers such as Dorothea Dix tried to persuade the federal government to expand its powers for the cause of the mentally ill. After she convinced state governments to pass legislation to help the insane, Dix began in 1850 to lobby Congress to pass a bill that would set aside 10 million acres of public lands in each of the states. The sale of these public lands would help support the mentally ill poor in the states. President Franklin Pierce, elected in 1852, did not share the reforming fervor of his fellow New Englander. He entered office as a supporter of a strict interpretation of the Constitution and believed that state and local government should be left in charge of the poor and disabled. Pierce decided not to sign the legislation and eventually vetoed it. In the following selection taken from his veto message to the Senate, Pierce explains that the proposed law violated his view of the proper relationship between state and federal government. He was also concerned that by making the federal government responsible for the insane, private charity of all kinds would be undermined.

To the Senate of the United States:

The bill entitled "An act making a grant of public lands [land owned by the federal government] to the several States for the benefit of indigent insane persons," which was presented to me on the 27th ultimo, has been maturely considered, and is returned to the Senate, the House in which it originated, with a statement of the objections which have required me to withhold from it my approval.

Franklin Pierce, "Veto Message, May 3, 1854," *A Compilation of the Messages and Papers of the Presidents, 1789–1897.* http://ksghome.harvard.edu/~phall/dochistcontents.html.

In the performance of this duty, prescribed by the Constitution, I have been compelled to resist the deep sympathies of my own heart in favor of the humane purpose sought to be accomplished and to overcome the reluctance with which I dissent from the conclusions of the two Houses of Congress, and present my own opinions in opposition to the action of a coordinate branch of the Government which possesses so fully my confidence and respect.

If in presenting my objections to this bill I should say more than strictly belongs to the measure or is required for the discharge of my official obligation, let it be attributed to a sincere desire to justify my act before those whose good opinion I so highly value and to that earnestness which springs from my deliberate conviction that a strict adherence to the terms and purposes of the federal compact offers the best, if not the only, security for the preservation of our blessed inheritance of representative liberty.

The bill provides in substance:

First. That 10,000,000 acres of land be granted to the several States, to be apportioned among them in the compound ratio of the geographical area and representation of said States in the House of Representatives.

Second. That wherever there are public lands in a State subject to sale at the regular price of private entry, the proportion of said 10,000,000 acres falling to such State shall be selected from such lands within it, and that to the States in which there are no such public lands land scrip shall be issued to the amount of their distributive shares [states where no public land was available would be issued title to land elsewhere], respectively, said scrip not to be entered by said States, but to be sold by them and subject to entry by their assignees: *Provided,* That none of it shall be sold at less than $1 per acre, under penalty of forfeiture of the same to the United States.

Third. That the expenses of the management and superintendence of said lands and of the moneys received therefrom shall be paid by the States to which they may belong out of the treasury of said States.

Fourth. That the gross proceeds of the sales of such lands or land scrip so granted shall be invested by the several States in safe stocks, to constitute a perpetual fund, the principal of which shall remain forever undiminished, and the interest to be appropriated to the maintenance of the indigent insane within the several States.

Fifth. That annual returns of lands or scrip sold shall be made by the States to the Secretary of the Interior, and the whole grant be subject to certain conditions and limitations prescribed in the bill, to be assented to by legislative acts of said States.

This bill therefore proposes that the Federal Government shall make provision to the amount of the value of 10,000,000 acres of land for an eleemosynary object [for charitable purposes] within the several States, to be administered by the political authority of the same; and it presents at the threshold the question whether any such act on the part of the Federal Government is warranted and sanctioned by the Constitution, the provisions and principles of which are to be protected and sustained as a first and paramount duty.

It cannot be questioned that if Congress has the power to make provision for the indigent insane without the limits of this District it has the same power to provide for the indigent who are not insane, and thus to transfer to the Federal Government the charger of all the poor in all the States. It has the same power to provide hospitals and other local establishments for the care and cure of every species of human infirmity, and thus to assume all that duty of either public philanthropy or public necessity to the dependent, the orphan, the sick, or the needy which is now discharged by the States themselves or by corporate institutions or private endowments existing under the legislation of the States. The whole field of public beneficence is thrown open to the care and culture of the Federal Government. Generous impulses no longer encounter the limitations and control of our imperious fundamental law; for however worthy may be the present object in itself, it is only one of a class. It is not exclusively worthy of benevolent regard. Whatever considerations dictate sympathy for this particular object apply in like manner, if not in the same degree, to idiocy, to physical disease, to extreme destitution. If Congress may and ought to provide for any one of these objects, it may and ought to provide for them all. And if it be done in this case, what answer shall be given when Congress shall be called upon, as it doubtless will be, to pursue a similar course of legislation in the others? It will obviously be vain to reply that the object is worthy, but that the application has taken a wrong direction. The power will have been deliberately assumed, the general obligation will by this act have been acknowledged, and the question of means and expediency will alone be left for consideration. The decision upon the principle in any one case determines it for the whole class. The question presented, therefore, clearly is upon the constitutionality and propriety of the Federal Government assuming to enter into a novel and vast field of legislation, namely, that of providing for the care and support of all those among the people of the United States who by any form become fit objects of public philanthropy.

Not the "Great Almoner"

I readily and, I trust, feelingly acknowledge the duty incumbent on us all as men and citizens, and as among the highest and holiest of our duties, to provide for those who, in the mysterious order of Providence, are subject to want and to disease of body or mind; but I can not find any authority in the Constitution for making the Federal Government the great almoner of public charity throughout the United States. To do so would, in my judgement, be contrary to the letter and spirit of the Constitution and subversive of the whole theory upon which the Union of these States is founded. And if it were admissible to contemplate the exercise of this power for any object whatever, I can not avoid the belief that it would in the end be prejudicial rather than beneficial to the noble offices of charity to have the charge of them transferred from the States to the Federal Government. Are we not too prone to forget that the Federal Union is the creature of the States, not they of the Federal Union? We were the inhabitants of colonies distinct in local government from one another before the Revolution. By the Revolution the colonies each became an independent State. They achieved that independence and secured its recognition by the agency of a consulting body, which, from being an assembly of the ministers of distinct sovereignties instructed to agree to no form of government which did not leave the domestic concerns of each State to itself, was appropriately denominated a Congress. When, having tried the experiment of the Confederation, they resolved to change that for the present Federal Union, and thus to confer on the Federal Government more ample authority, they scrupulously measured such of the functions of their cherished sovereignty as they chose to delegate to the General Government. With the aim and to this end the fathers of the Republic framed the Constitution, in and by which the independent and sovereign States united themselves for certain specified objects and purposes, and for those only, leaving all powers not therein set forth as conferred on one or another of the great departments—the legislative, the executive, and the judicial—indubitably within the States. And when the people of the several States had in their State conventions, and thus alone, given effect and force to the Constitution, not content that any doubt should in the future arise as to the scope and character of this act, they ingrafted thereon the explicit declaration that "the powers not delegated to the United States by the Constitution nor prohibited by it to the States are reserved to the States respectively or to the people."...

The framers of the Constitution, ... in my judgement manifested a wise forecast and broad comprehension of the true interests of these objects themselves. It is clear that public charities within the States can be efficiently administered only by their authority. The bill before me concedes this, for it does not commit funds it provides to the administration of any other authority.

I can not but repeat what I have before expressed, that if the several States, many of which have already laid the foundation of munificent establishments of local beneficence, and nearly all of which are proceeding to establish them, shall be led to suppose, as, should this bill become a law, they will be, that Congress is to make provision for such objects, the fountains of charity will be dried up at home, and the several States, instead of bestowing their own means on the social wants of their own people, may themselves, through the strong temptation which appeals to the states as to individuals, become humble suppliants for the bounty of the Federal Government, reversing their true relations to this Union....

To Dispose of the Public Domain

To assume that the public lands are applicable to ordinary State objects, whether of public structures, police, charity, or expenses of State administration, would be to disregard to the amount of the value of the public lands, all the limitations of the Constitution and confound to that extend all distinctions between the rights and powers of the States and those of the United States; for if the public lands may be applied to the support of the poor, whether sane or insane, if the disposal of them and their proceeds be not subject to the ordinary limitations of the Constitution, then Congress possesses unqualified power to provide for expenditures in the States by means of the public lands, even to the degree of defraying the salaries of governors, judges, and all other expenses of the government and internal administration within the several States.

The conclusion from the general survey of the whole subject is to my mind irresistible, and closes the question both of right and expediency so far as regards the principle of the appropriation proposed in this bill. Would not the admission of such power in Congress to dispose of the public domain work the practical abrogation of some of the most important provisions of the Constitution?

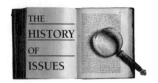

CHAPTER 2

The Era of
Mental Institutions

Chapter Preface

The opening of Pennsylvania Hospital in 1751 inaugurated a new era in the treatment of the mentally ill in the United States. Founded by Dr. Thomas Bond and Benjamin Franklin, Pennsylvania Hospital began by taking in individuals suffering from mental illness and attempting to treat them using the medical techniques of the day. Gradually, the hospital was transformed into one of the first of a new kind of institution, one that would dominate mental health care well into the twentieth century: the insane asylum.

Asylums in America followed the example of mental health-care pioneer Philippe Pinel who, in 1793 removed the restraining chains of the mentally ill in his Parisian hospital. Pinel believed in the concept of psychological therapy and advocated kind, humane treatment of the insane in an environment that would lead to improvements in their conditions. Pinel's approach was called moral treatment or moral management in the United States where it was adopted by physicians such as Thomas Kirkbride.

In mid-nineteenth-century America the insane asylum, particularly those organized along the principles of Thomas Kirkbride, was regarded as the symbol of an enlightened and progressive nation. Asylums fulfilled many needs: They benefited the community, the family, and the individual by offering the most effective medical treatment available for the severely ill and humane custodial care for chronic cases. By building asylums and providing for persons with mental illness, state governments met their ethical and moral responsibilities and contributed to the general welfare of the populace, states noted historian Gerald N. Grob. Within the asylum, patients were isolated from the stressors of society and lived in a well-organized environment with a gentle and firm daily routine. All of these aspects were seen as beneficial and helpful in restoring a person to health.

By the late 1800s, however, the asylums—now called state hospitals—had become victims of their own success. They were sent not just the mentally ill, but all those who were too poor and unhealthy to take care of themselves. In addition to their responsibilities for curing the mentally ill, doctors and staff became custodians of those who required long-term care. Overcrowding and lack of funding in subsequent decades led to a stagnation and decline in the quality of care. By the mid-1940s the mental asylum came to be regarded as a dinosaur, a remnant of a previous era, and worse, a dumping ground for the least fortunate of society. Reformers called for drastic changes in the way state hospitals functioned and demanded that the least effective be shut down. This chapter presents the history of the mental asylum, which began as a bold reform in mental health care but would come to be seen as a failure in need of reform in its own right.

Hospitalization of the Mentally Ill: The Pennsylvania Hospital Is Founded

Thomas Morton

In 1751 Benjamin Franklin and Dr. Thomas Bond established a hospital in Philadelphia for the purpose of caring for "the sick-poor and insane who were wandering the streets of Philadelphia." Pennsylvania Hospital was the first hospital in the American colonies. At the time, Philadelphia was the fastest growing city in the American colonies and had a population of approximately fifteen thousand. It was a major port with a multifaceted populace: the rich and poor coexisted alongside a growing number of immigrant workers. Bond, a Quaker, saw the need for an institution that would help Philadelphians of all economic classes who were suffering from physical and mental disease. Benjamin Franklin, a friend of Bond's, supported the idea and organized a petition to the Pennsylvania Assembly. When the assembly seemed less than enthusiastic, Franklin offered to raise two thousand pounds from private citizens. If he could accomplish this, then the assembly would match the funds with an additional two thousand pounds. All funds were raised and in 1751 the plan to build Pennsylvania Hospital was signed into law by the colonial governor.

In the following decades Pennsylvania Hospital became the model for mental asylums in the United States. The following selection is taken from a history of the hospital written in 1895 by one of its leading doctors, Thomas Morton. In it, Morton lists the general rules of the Department of the Insane as they pertained to the physician in chief, his staff, the patients, and visitors. In the 1890s the hospital was no longer solely a charitable institution and admitted only a specific number of poor patients

Thomas Morton, *The History of the Pennsylvania Hospital, 1751–1895*, Philadelphia: Times Printing House, 1895, pp. 559–562.

who had a reasonable chance of recovery. All other patients paid board based on their financial situations.

The officers of the Pennsylvania Hospital Department for the Insane, shall consist of a Physician-in-Chief and Superintendent, for the whole establishment, and one or more Assistant Physicians, also a consulting Gynecologist, and a Steward and a Matron for each department.

The Physician-in-Chief

1. The Physician-in-Chief and Superintendent of the Hospital for the Insane, shall be the official head of that department; and, under the instructions of the Board of Managers, shall have the general superintendence and control thereof and of all persons employed on the premises.

2. He shall reside upon the premises, and devote his whole time to the promotion of the interests of the Institution and the welfare and comfort of the patients.

3. He shall have the sole direction of the medical, moral, and dietetic treatment of the patients, and his directions respecting them are to be implicitly obeyed by all persons about the establishment.

4. He shall have the power to select and dismiss at his pleasure all the attendants and other persons employed in the care of the Insane, and the sole direction of their duties. With the sanction of the Attending Managers, he shall from time to time make such regulations for the government of the attendants, and all others engaged in any way about the Institution, as he may deem salutary.

5. He shall have the general direction of the farm, gardens, and grounds of the Hospital; and may make contracts with the farmer and others employed thereon, and with the tenants, (subject to approval by the Board of Managers).

6. He shall obtain as far as practicable, a complete history of the case of every patient admitted into the Hospital, and

shall keep or cause to be kept, for the use of the Institution, a register of the same, and as full a record of the subsequent treatment and results as he may deem likely to promote the interests of science, and tend to improve the treatment of the insane.

7. He shall furnish to the Board of Managers annually, at its stated meeting in the fourth month (April) in each year, a detailed report of the operations of the Hospital, with tabular statements of the cases treated during the preceding twelve months, and of its actual condition; with such other observations as he may deem useful or interesting.

8. All correspondence respecting the patients, shall be under his direction.

9. He shall exercise a vigilant supervision of all expenditures, and as far as he can, shall indicate by some mark on all bills or receipts, that no purchases have been made or expenses incurred without his approval, or at least without his knowledge.

The Assistant Physicians

1. The Assistant Physician shall reside in the Hospital and, under the direction of the Physician-in-Chief and Superintendent, shall devote their whole time to its service, and carry out to the best of their abilities, all the instructions of that officer.

2. They shall prepare and superintend the administration of all medicines prescribed for the patients; preserving in a book provided for the purpose, every prescription, with the name of the patient, and shall keep or assist in keeping such records, and performing such other duties as may be required by the Physician-in-Chief and Superintendent.

3. They shall be as much as possible among the patients, visiting them regularly every morning and evening, and as often as they can at other hours, and do all in their power to contribute to their comfort and welfare, they shall have a gen-

eral supervision of the attendants, and shall promptly report to the Physician-in-Chief and Superintendent, all instances of neglect or of improper conduct on the part of any one connected with the Institution, that may come to their knowledge.

4. It shall also be the duty of one of the Assistant Physicians to attend at the Out-Patient Department on Pine Street for consultation on Mental and Nervous diseases.

5. They shall not absent themselves from the Hospital without the knowledge and consent of the Physician-in-Chief and Superintendent, and the Attending Managers.

The Stewards

1. Under the instructions of the Physician-in-Chief and Superintendent, the Stewards shall have a general oversight of the buildings, grounds, and farm and shall see that they are at all times kept in perfect order and repair, and that all persons employed about the same perform their duties faithfully.

2. Under the direction of the Physician-in-Chief and Superintendent and subject to the instructions of the Attending Managers, they shall purchase furniture, fuel, clothing, stores, and all other necessary articles, and shall be responsible for their safe keeping and economical use.

3. They shall collect all moneys due the Institution for board of patients, etc., as they become due, and shall keep plain and accurate accounts of the receipts and expenditures. They shall furnish transcripts thereof, approved by the Attending Managers, to be laid before the Board at each of their stated meetings. They shall also keep a regular register of the names and of the dates admission and discharge of every patient.

4. Subject to the authority given to the Physician-in-Chief and Superintendent, and under his instructions, they shall hire, pay, and discharge all persons employed about the premises.

5. They shall pay particular attention to the quality of the provisions provided for the use of the Institution, and the manner in which they are cooked and served. They shall visit the dining-rooms during meals, and see that all things appertaining to them are disposed in a neat and becoming manner, that good order and perfect cleanliness are preserved in every part of the house coming under their notice, shall promptly report to the Physician-in-Chief and Superintendent all instances of neglect or improper conduct that they may observe, and, as far as practicable, see that the warming and ventilation of the buildings are properly regulated.

The Matrons

It shall be the duty of the matrons to have the immediate charge of the housekeeping. They shall observe the manner in which the attendants and other perform their duties and report to the Physician-in-Chief and Superintendent any instance of neglect or improper conduct coming under their notice. They shall have general oversight and direction of the domestics, and shall superintend and direct the cooking and distribution of food, and, in conjunction with the Stewards, shall see that the supply is abundant, varied, well-cooked, and neatly served, in all the dining-rooms of the establishment, which they shall visit as often as possible at the hours for meals. They shall also see that the bedding, clothing, etc., of the patients are always kept clean and in good order. They are expected to devote their whole time to the service of the Institution, and under the instructions of the Physician-in-Chief and Superintendent, to spare no efforts to promote its prosperity.

General Rules

All persons engaged, in any way, about the Institution, shall be careful to conform to the regulations made for the government of the Hospital, and at all times do what they can to promote its prosperity. No smoking of tobacco by any thus employed, shall be allowed within the enclosures, nor in the vicinity of the barns or other outbuildings; nor shall any persons be employed who are addicted to the use of spirituous liquors.

All lights, except in the wards, entries, Steward's Matron's Physicians' rooms, are required to be extinguished at ten o'clock P.M. No reading in bed at night is to be allowed, either by patients or by any person connected with the establishment in any capacity.

Admission of Patients

1. Before any patient can be admitted into this Hospital, a request in writing to that effect from some near relative or friend, and a certificate of said patient's insanity, signed by two respectable graduates of medicine, shall in all cases be required, in the mode prescribed by the laws of Pennsylvania.

2. Neither idiots nor persons having mania-à-potû [madness due to chronic drinking], shall be received into this Hospital.

3. A limited number of insane persons in indigents circumstances, whose cases are recent, and such as are believed to offer a fair chance of cure, shall be admitted as patients by the Attending Managers, for a period not exceeding three months for each case, and shall be treated without any charge. If promising favorably, and on the recommendation of the Physician-in-Chief and Superintendent, the period may be extended at the discretion of the Board. Security for the removal of such patients when discharged, and for their clothing whilst in the Hospital, shall be required of some responsible resident of the city of Philadelphia, or its vicinity. The number of these patients shall from time to time be regulated by the Board of Managers, and is now fixed at fifty.

4. Patients paying board may be admitted by any member of the Board of Managers, under the following rules.

5. The rate of board shall be regulated by the pecuniary ability of the patient, or of the friends of the patient, and the class of accommodations required. The lowest rate shall be nine dollars per week. They shall not be admitted for a less period than three months, for which time the board shall be required to be paid in advance at the time of admission; and if taken away *uncured* before the expiration of that period, contrary to the advice and consent of the Physician-in-Chief and Superintendent of the Hospital, the amount as above paid in advance shall be considered forfeited, and no part thereof shall be returned. Four weeks' board shall be retained in all cases. All payments shall be made quarterly in advance. Security of some responsible resident of the city of Philadelphia, or its vicinity, shall in all cases obtained, for the payment of board and all other expenses whilst in the institution, and for the performance of the foregoing conditions.

6. When special attendants are desired they are always to be provided by the Physician of the Hospital, and the charge therefor to be added to the board.

Admission of Visitors

The Board of Managers—recognizing the duty of shielding the insane from all improper exposure, and regarding their right of protection from the gratification of an idle curiosity on the part of strangers just as great, while residents of a hospital, as in their own dwellings—have adopted the following regulations for the admission of visitors:

1. Visitors are not to be admitted before 10 o'clock A.M., after sunset, nor on the First day of the week. They are not to be admitted on the afternoon of Seventh day (Saturday) unless on special business with the Attending Managers, or one of the officers of the house.

2. All parts of the Hospital *not occupied by patients* may be shown and explained during the hours for the admission of visitors.

3. No visitors, unless in company with a Manager, can be taken into the wards, without permission from the Physician-in-Chief, or, in his absence, from an Assistant Physician; and when visitors are allowed in the wards, they must always be accompanied by one of these officers, by the Steward or Matron, or by some person delegated by the Physician for the purpose.

4. As this Hospital cannot be allowed to become a resort for idle curiosity, it is hoped that the friends patients, and all others, will carefully avoid prolonging their visits unnecessarily. And those employed in the care of patients, or in the domestic departments, are to avoid inviting company to the Hospital.

5. The Pleasure Carriages and other contrivances for the amusement of patients, are not to be used by visitors; nor are they to enter the museums or to pass through the pleasure grounds, except by special permission.

6. It is expressly forbidden to furnish any inmate of this Hospital with tobacco in any form; or to deliver to, or receive from a patient, any letter, parcel, or package, without the knowledge and approbation of the Physician.

7. Funds for the use of the patients are to be placed in the hands of the Stewards, to be used only under the direction of the Physician.

8. Under ordinary circumstances, carriages are not to enter the enclosures. When for any purpose they have been taken to the centre buildings, they are never to be left standing there; and drivers are always expected to remain with their vehicles outside of the gateway.

Thomas Kirkbride and "Asylum Medicine"

Nancy Tomes

In 1841 Pennsylvania Hospital opened a second facility called the Pennsylvania Hospital for the Insane. One of the leading physicians in the history of the treatment of the mentally ill in the United States, Thomas Story Kirkbride (1809–1883) served as chief physician of the new facility from 1841 until his death forty-three years later. Kirkbride, a Quaker, believed in the "moral treatment" of the mentally ill. This meant treating the ill with compassion and respect in a physical setting that was constructed to calm and refresh them. In keeping with this philosophy, Kirkbride designed an attractive, rambling building for his hospital that was set amidst pleasant grounds and isolated from the energy of the city. As described by author Nancy Tomes in the following selection from her book on Kirkbride, the goal of the physican in chief of the asylum was twofold: to provide a comfortable, homelike surrounding for patients and to control and manage them in a secure setting. Over time, the so-called Kirkbride plan for mental asylums became the model for state asylums built in such cities as Trenton, New Jersey; Worcester, Massachusetts; and Buffalo, New York. By the early 1900s, however, the concept of building as cure was discarded and the large, Victorian-style buildings set on acres of open land were regarded as too expensive to maintain. Many fell into disuse and were eventually closed down while others were renovated for other uses.

Upon arriving at the Pennsylvania Hospital [for the Insane] after a long carriage ride from the city, the families of prospective patients beheld an institution quite unlike the

Nancy Tomes, *The Art of Asylum-Keeping: Thomas Kirkbride and the Origins of American Psychiatry*, Philadelphia: University of Pennsylvania Press, 1984, pp. 129–130, 132, 134, 140–146. Paperback reprint edition copyright © 1994 by Nancy Tomes. All rights reserved. Reprinted by permission of the University of Pennsylvania Press.

horrible madhouse they had feared. Its secluded rural location promised the protection from public notoriety they desired, and the pleasant, even luxurious appearance of the building and grounds belied grim preconceptions of institutional life. Wherever the patrons looked, from the ten-pin bowling alley to the reading room, they saw evidence of the efforts made to watch over and amuse the patients, efforts far more extensive and well organized than their own home regimen. Meeting the asylum superintendent, who spoke to them with a blend of paternal concern and scientific authority, the family found themselves further comforted. From first to last, every aspect of the asylum's appearance and organization seemed designed expressly to relieve and reassure them. The institution and, more importantly, the physician at its head held out to the family the promise of a benign control, a persuasive influence, that would rid insanity of its horrors.

The impressions created by the Pennsylvania Hospital for the Insane were hardly effortless or unpremeditated. The reassuring details of its regimen and appearance reflected Thomas Story Kirkbride's painstaking labor. From his earliest years as superintendent, he made the creation and maintenance of the asylum's therapeutic image his central professional concern. Personal factors, including his father's pursuit of agricultural improvements and his own practical bent, so early manifested in the love of surgery, contributed to Kirkbride's interest in asylum construction. His devotion to the [Society of] Friends' principles no doubt made him particularly sensitive to the sufferings caused by insanity and desirous of relieving them. All these predilections found expression in Kirkbride's philosophy of asylum medicine, which made hospital design and administration central to its practice. This philosophy, first enunciated in an 1847 article in the *American Journal of Medical Science* and then amplified in his 1854 book, *On the Construction, Management, and General Arrangements of Hospitals for the Insane,* not only guided Kirkbride's own practice at the

Pennsylvania Hospital for the Insane but became the dominant credo for the whole American specialty.

More than any of his contemporaries, Kirkbride divined the importance of institutional forms to the profession's success. The moral architecture and moral order of the new hospital, he realized, were the most powerful means physicians possessed to summon up belief in the new asylum treatment. The asylum doctors' reputation as healers of mental disease depended almost entirely on their ability to inspire faith in this, their most impressive asset: the mental hospital. To extend medical jurisdiction over insanity, Kirkbride developed an asylum philosophy designed to control the hospital environment completely. Every detail, from the design of the window frames to the table settings in the ward dining rooms, had to be arranged to sustain the impression that here was an institution where patients received kind and competent care. . . .

Kirkbride's Reports

The dominant elements of Kirkbride's therapeutic persuasion can be traced most clearly in his *Reports of the Pennsylvania Hospital for the Insane*, which he published annually. Although written for several audiences, including his managers, professional brethren, and potential contributors, Kirkbride's *Reports* functioned primarily as brochures designed to attract and inform readers who might be considering asylum treatment for an insane relative or friend. . . .

In addition to spelling out the terms of admission to the Pennsylvania Hospital for the Insane, the *Reports* provided elementary information about the nature of insanity. Kirkbride defined insanity simply as a "functional disease of the brain" and offered no detailed discussion of its pathology, preferring instead to elaborate on the proper attitude to be taken toward the disease. Couched in soothing, nonjudgmental terms, his explanations presented insanity as a disease that might affect anyone. "Insanity is truly the great leveler of all the artificial distinctions of society," he frequently told his readers. He minimized the sufferer's personal responsibility for the disease, characterizing it as "an accident . . . to which we are all liable, and especially, if without any direct agency of our own, or certainly without anything on our part that was dishonorable or criminal . . . no reproach to anyone." (Note the use of the inclusive pronoun.) Although "prudence and a good constitution" might successfully ward off mental disease, even respectable, morally irreproachable people might be stricken with it; "it is found among the purest and the best of all dwellers upon earth, as well as those who are far from being models of excellence," he wrote. Kirkbride also denied that heredity played a major role in most mental disease. Feeling that medical and lay thinking accorded too much importance to hereditary propensities, he urged the families of the insane not to scrutinize anxiously all their relatives for signs of some ancestral taint. . . .

To Reassure the Public

Kirkbride projected a reassuring set of beliefs about insanity and hospital treatment, beliefs that helped families and friends make sense of the disease and encouraged their patronage of the hospital. Kirkbride had to do more than simply explain these truths in the *Reports*, however. The asylum itself had to confirm his arguments whenever family members came to commit a patient or returned to visit. By comparing the image of the hospital created in his *Reports* with his professional writings on asylum construction and management, it becomes clear how the desire to impress and reassure his lay patrons shaped Kirkbride's professional priorities. From the perspective of his lay clientele, his attention to particular aspects of the hospital's appearance and function takes on new significance. One can begin to see how he worked to have the building's design and organization reinforce his patrons' beliefs about the hospital and eliminate certain realities of institutional life that might potentially undermine such confidence. . . .

Kirkbride's concern with asylum construction began literally from the ground up, with the choice of a good site. He advised that the hospital be located outside a city of some size, and easily accessible by train and good roads. Such a location would ensure plentiful supplies and employees, as well as varied excursions for the patients. The hospital itself, he instructed, should be in a secluded area to ensure complete privacy. The soil had to be easily tilled, so that the farm and gardens would produce food for the patients' table and the area around the hospital itself could be extensively improved. "The surrounding scenery should be of a varied and attractive kind, and the neighborhood should possess numerous objects of an agreeable and interesting character," he wrote. The building itself should be placed so that the views from every window, especially the parlors and rooms occupied during the day, had pleasant prospects and "exhibit[ed] life in its active forms." The choice of a good site thus determined some of the hospital's most desirable features in its patrons' eyes: its accessibility, attractiveness, and supply of fresh food.

The advantages of a good site had to be complemented by a sound building design. The general layout of the hospital determined two vital aspects of institutional life: the internal environment of the building, particularly its lighting and ventilation, and the proper classification of patients. The linear, or Kirkbride, plan, as set forth in his 1854 treatise, emphasized several important features as fundamental to a good building plan. It had wings radiating off the center section . . . so that each ward had proper ventilation and an unobstructed view of the grounds. By leaving open spaces at the end of each wing, "the darkest, most cheerless and worst ventilated parts" of the hospital could be eliminated, Kirkbride explained. He also advised inserting bay windows in the long halls, so that more light and air could enter. If the wings were not close together, there was "less opportunity for patients on opposite sides seeing or calling to each other, and less probability of the quiet patients being disturbed by those who are noisy." The linear plan also allowed for the maximum separation of the wards, so that the undesirable mingling of the patients might be prevented. Male and female patients had entirely separate wings. Within the wing, each ward had its own staircase, so that the patients might proceed directly outside to the pleasure grounds or to the center building without marching through another ward. Eight wards, the minimum Kirkbride felt desirable, could be established in each wing. He advised that the worst patients be confined in the ground-floor wards farthest from the center building and the best patients in the top-floor wards closer to the center. "A classification that admits of no greater mingling of patients than this," Kirkbride concluded, "is quite rigid for all practical purposes."

The style as well as the layout of the building had to be carefully considered. "Although it is not desirable to have an elaborate or costly style of architecture," Kirkbride wrote, "it is, nevertheless, really important that the building should be in good taste, and that it should impress favorably not only the patients, but their friends and others who may visit it." Any resemblance to a prison had to be carefully avoided. "The means of effecting the proper degree of security should be masked," he advised, and the building's custodial appearance camouflaged by ornamenting its grounds with gardens, fountains, and summer houses. These external improvements cost a considerable amount of money, Kirkbride acknowledged, but played such an important role in convincing patients and their families to support the institution that they could not be neglected. Every detail made a difference, he warned, for "no one can tell how important all these may prove in the treatment of patients, nor what good effects may result from first impressions thus made upon an invalid on reaching a hospital."

The good impression made by the building's exterior arrangements had to be sustained by the appearance and practicality of its interior. "No desire to make a beautiful and picturesque exterior should ever be allowed to interfere with the internal arrangements," Kirbride wrote. The interior had to sustain the cheerfulness of its exterior; as he advised one asylum superintendent, "have your parlors and rooms large and airy, with high ceilings, your corridors wide," and the overall good impression of the building would be sustained.

Balancing the need to make the building appear as inviting as possible with the imperative to provide adequate restraint for its inmates posed the most difficult challenge Kirkbride faced in asylum design. Security measures inevitably detracted from the attractive image Kirkbride wished the hospital to have; yet, he felt the patient safety had to be the chief priority in its arrangements. As he wrote to Dorothea Dix in 1856, "The death of a single patient in ten years, or the escape and public suffering of one insane man or woman, would be a greater evil, than all the properly constructed window guards to be found about a well arranged Hospital." Only by painstaking attention to details, Kirkbride believed, could the asylum be made secure without taking on the features of a prison. To this end, he showed considerable ingenuity in making the asylum's measures of restraint as unobtrusive as possible.

For example, Kirkbride believed that a mental hospital had to have a high wall around it to keep patients from escaping; at the same time, he did not want an obtrusive enclosure that would constantly remind visitors and patients of its confining purpose. As a compromise, Kirkbride proposed putting the wall as far from the building as possible, even sinking it in a trench, "to prevent its being an unpleasant feature, or to give the idea of a prison enclosure." He also attempted to soften the forbidding aspects of the wall by pointing out that it sheltered as well as confined the patients "by keeping improper persons out, by securing complete privacy to the institution," and by "protecting [patients] while out of the wards from the unfeeling gaze and remarks of passers by."

Careful construction of the building's interior further minimized the potential for disruptive events in the hospital. Many of Kirkbride's detailed designs for ward fixtures reveal his underlying concern with the prevention of destruction, violence, suicide, and escape. Doors should always be made to open into the hallway, he advised, "as great annoyance and no little danger frequently results from patients barricading their doors from the inside, so as to render it almost impossible to get access to them." "Wickets" should be put in the doors so that patients could be observed or given food "when it might not be prudent for a single individual to enter the room." In constructing windows, the lower sash should be protected by a wrought iron window guard, so that it could be opened to admit air without allowing the patient to escape. This guard, "if properly made, and painted a white color, will not prove unsightly," unlike a cast iron sash, which, when raised, gave the appearance of "two sets of iron bars." A window guard "of tasteful pattern and neatly made" appeared no more forbidding than the devices used in the front windows "of some of the best houses in our large cities," Kirkbride claimed. . . .

In the section of the building designed for less destructive patients, Kirkbride concentrated on making the wards as attractive and comfortable as possible. In order to convince patients and their families that hospital treatment involved no hardships, the wards had to appear homelike. The inevitable smells of an institution formed one of the biggest obstacles in this respect. Kirkbride's concern with ventilation originated in this practical problem. A good system of forced-air ventilation was "indispensable to give purity to the air of a hospital for the insane," he felt. . . .

These examples demonstrate the ways in which Kirkbride related design and construction details to the asylum image he created in the *Reports*. In a properly constructed hospital, so he hoped, no escapes, suicides, and offensive smells would dis-turb either the patients or their families.

A Memoir of an Illness

Clifford Whittingham Beers

Up until the early 1900s descriptions of mental illness had largely been the domain of physicians such as Thomas Kirkbride, chief physician of the Pennsylvania Hospital for the Insane, or reformers such as Dorothea Dix. Clifford Whittingham Beers (1876–1943) wrote a personal account of what it was like to suffer a mental breakdown, experience commitment to an asylum, and recover one's health. His autobiography, A Mind That Found Itself, *was first published in 1907.*

A native of New Haven, Connecticut, and a recent graduate of Yale University, Beers suffered a nervous collapse and attempted suicide in 1900. This event resulted in his commitment to the first of several mental asylums. After three years of hospitalization, Beers regained his health and went on to write about his experiences in the hospitals where he was confined and treated. An excerpt from his autobiography is included here. Beers' story of the abuses he suffered in the hospitals, such as being straitjacketed and beaten by attendants, gained him the attention of psychiatrist Dr. Adolph Meyer and psychologist William James. They put him in contact with others who saw the need to reform mental hospitals and educate the public about mental illness. With their support Beers established the National Committee for Mental Hygiene, the first organization that, among other accomplishments, published statistical reports about mental illness, helped develop psychiatric training curricula, and worked to prevent mental illness and the need for hospitalization. Most importantly, Beers and his organization urged legislators to fund an enlarged mental health service system.

On the thirtieth day of June, 1897, I graduated at Yale. Had I then realized that I was a sick man, I could and would have taken a rest. But, in a way, I had become accustomed to the ups and downs of a nervous existence, and, as I could not really afford a rest, six days after my graduation I entered upon the duties of a clerk in the office of the Collector of Taxes in the city of New Haven. I was fortunate in securing such a position at that time, for the hours were comparatively short and the work as congenial as any could have been under the circumstances. I entered the Tax Office with the intention of staying only until such time as I might secure a position in New York. About a year later I secured the desired position. After remaining in it for eight months I left it, in order to take a position which seemed to offer a field of endeavor more to my taste. From May, 1899, till the middle of June, 1900, I was a clerk in one of the smaller life-insurance companies, whose home office was within a stone's throw of what some men consider the center of the universe. To be in the very heart of the financial district of New York appealed strongly to my imagination. As a result of the contagious ideals of Wall Street, the making of money was then a passion with me. I wished to taste the bitter-sweet of power based on wealth.

For the first eighteen months of my life in New York, my health seemed no worse than it had been during the preceding three years. But the old dread still possessed me. I continued to have my more and less nervous days, weeks, and months. In March, 1900, however, there came a change for the worse. At that time I had a severe attack of grippe [influenza, or a similar disease] which incapacitated me for two weeks. As was to be expected in my case, this illness seriously depleted my vitality, and left me in a frightfully depressed condition—a depression which continued to grow upon me until the final crash came, on June 23rd, 1900. The events of that day, seemingly disastrous as then viewed, but evidently all for the best as the issue proved, forced me along paths traveled by thousands, but comprehended by few.

I had continued to perform my clerical duties until June 15th. On that day I was compelled to stop, and that at once. I had reached a point where my will had to capitulate to Unreason—that unscrupulous usurper. My previous five years as a neurasthenic [someone who suffers from chronic fatigue] had led me to believe that I had experienced all the disagreeable sensations an overworked and unstrung nervous system could suffer. But on this day several new and terrifying sensations seized me and rendered me all but helpless. My condition, however, was not apparent even to those who worked with me at the same desk. I remember trying to speak and at times finding myself unable to give utterance to my thoughts. Though I was able to answer questions, that fact hardly diminished my feeling of apprehension, for a single failure in an attempt to speak will stagger any man, no matter what his state of health. I tried to copy certain records in the day's work, but my hand was too unsteady, and I found it difficult to read the words and figures presented to my tired vision in blurred confusion.

That afternoon, conscious that some terrible calamity was impending, but not knowing what would be its nature, I performed a very curious act. Certain early literary efforts which had failed of publication in the college paper, but which I had jealously cherished for several years, I utterly destroyed. Then, after a hurried arrangement of my affairs, I took an early afternoon train, and was soon in New Haven. Home life did not make me better, and, except for three or four short walks, I did not go out of the house at all until June 23d, when I went in a most unusual way. To relatives I said little about my state of health, beyond the general statement that I had never felt worse—a statement which, when made by a neurasthenic, means much, but proves little. For five years I had had my ups and downs, and both my relatives and myself had begun to look upon these as things which would probably be corrected in and by time.

A Delusion

The day after my home-coming I made up my mind, or that part of it which was still within my control, that the time had come to quit business entirely and take a rest of months. I even arranged with a younger brother to set out at once for some quiet place in the White Mountains, where I hoped to steady my shattered nerves. At this time I felt as though in a tremor from head to foot, and the thought that I was about to have an epileptic attack constantly recurred. On more than one occasion I said to friends that I would rather die than live an epileptic; yet, if I rightly remember, I never declared the actual fear that I was doomed to bear such an affliction. Though I held the mad belief that I should suffer epilepsy, I held the sane hope, amounting to belief, that I should escape it. This fact may account, in a measure, for my six years of endurance.

On the 18th of June I felt so much worse that I went to my bed and stayed there until the 23d. During the night of the 18th my persistent dread became a false belief—a delusion. What I had long expected I now became convinced had at last occurred. I believed myself to be a confirmed epileptic, and that conviction was stronger than any ever held by a sound intellect. The half-resolve, made before my mind was actually impaired, namely, that I would kill myself rather than live the life I dreaded, now divided my attention with the belief that the stroke had fallen. From that time my one thought was to hasten the end, for I felt that I should lose the chance to die should relatives find me in an attack of epilepsy.

Considering the state of my mind and my inability at that time to appreciate the enormity of such an end as I half contemplated, my suicidal purpose was not entirely selfish. That I had never seriously contemplated suicide is proved by the fact that I had not provided myself with the means of accomplishing it, despite my habit, which has long been remarked by my friends, of preparing even for unlikely contingencies. So far as I had the control of my faculties, it must be admitted that I deliberated; but, strictly speaking, the rash act which followed cannot correctly be called an attempt at suicide—for how can a man who is not himself kill himself?

Soon my disordered brain was busy with schemes for death. I distinctly remember one which included a row on Lake Whitney, near New Haven. This I intended to take in the most unstable boat obtainable. Such a craft could be easily upset, and I should so bequeath to relatives and friends a sufficient number of reasonable doubts to rob my death of the usual stigma. I also remember searching for some deadly drug which I hoped to find about the house. But the quantity and quality of what I found were not such as I dared to trust. I then thought of severing my jugular vein, even going so far as to test against my throat the edge of a razor which, after the deadly impulse first asserted itself, I had secreted in a convenient place. I really wished to die, but so uncertain and ghastly a method did not appeal to me. Nevertheless, had I felt sure that in my tremulous frenzy I could accomplish the act with skillful dispatch, I should at once have ended my troubles.

My imaginary attacks were now recurring with distracting frequency, and I was in constant fear of discovery. During these three or four days I slept scarcely at all—even the medicine given to induce sleep having little effect. Though inwardly frenzied, I gave no outward sign of my condition. Most of the time I remained quietly in bed. I spoke but seldom. I had practically, though not entirely, lost the power of speech; but my almost unbroken silence aroused no suspicions as to the seriousness of my condition.

A Brain in Ferment

By a process of elimination, all suicidal methods but one had at last been put aside. On that one my mind now centered. My room was on the fourth floor of the house—one of a block of five—in which my parents lived. The house stood several feet back from the street. The sills of my windows were a little more than thirty feet above the ground. Under one was a flag pavement, extending from the house to the front gate. Under the other was a rectangular coal-hole covered with an iron grating. This was surrounded by flagging over a foot in width; and connecting it and the pavement proper was another flag. So that all along the front of the house, stone or iron filled a space at no point less than two feet in width. It required little calculation to determine how slight the chance of surviving a fall from either of those two windows.

About dawn I arose. Stealthily I approached a window, pushed open the blinds, and looked out—and down. Then I closed the blinds as noiselessly as possible and crept back to bed: I had not yet become so irresponsible that I dared to take the leap. Scarcely had I pulled up the covering when a watchful relative entered my room, drawn thither perhaps by that protecting prescience which love inspires. I thought her words revealed a suspicion that she had heard me at the window, but speechless as I was I had enough speech to deceive her. For of what account are Truth and Love when Life itself has ceased to seem desirable?

The dawn soon hid itself in the brilliancy of a perfect June day. Never had I seen a brighter—to look at; never a darker—to live through—or a better to die upon. Its very perfection and the songs of the robins, which at that season were plentiful in the neighborhood, served but to increase my despair and make me the more willing to die. As the day wore on, my anguish became more intense, but I managed to mislead those about me by uttering a word now and then, and feigning to read a newspaper, which to me, however, appeared an unintelligible jumble of type. My brain was in a ferment. It felt as if pricked by a million needles at white heat. My whole body felt as though it would be torn apart by the terrific nervous strain under which I labored.

Shortly after noon, dinner having been served, my mother entered the room and asked me if she should bring me some dessert. I assented. It was not that I cared for the dessert; I had no appetite. I wished to get her out of the room, for I believed myself to be on the verge of another attack. She left at once. I knew that in two or three minutes she would return. The crisis seemed at hand. It was now or never for liberation. She had probably descended one of three flights of stairs when, with the mad desire to dash my brains out on the pavement below, I rushed to that window which was directly over the flag walk. Providence must have guided my movements, for in some otherwise unaccountable way, on the very point of hurling myself out bodily, I chose to drop feet foremost instead. With my fingers I clung for a moment to the sill. Then I let go. In falling my body turned so as to bring my right side toward the building. I struck the ground a little more than two feet from the foundation of the house, and at least three to the left of the point from which I started. Missing the stone pavement by not more than three or four inches, I struck on comparatively soft earth. My position must have been almost upright, for both heels struck the ground squarely. The concussion slightly crushed one heel bone and broke most of the small bones in the arch of each foot, but there was no mutilation of the flesh. As my feet struck the ground my right hand struck hard against the front of the house, and it is probable that these three points of contact, dividing the force of the shock, prevented my back from being broken. As it was, it narrowly escaped a fracture and, for several weeks afterward, it felt as if powdered glass had been substituted for cartilage between the vertebræ.

I did not lose consciousness even for a second, and the demoniacal dread, which had possessed me from June, 1894, until this fall to earth just six years later, was dispelled the instant I struck the ground. At no time since have I experienced one of my imaginary attacks; nor has my mind even for a moment entertained such an idea. The little demon which had tortured me relentlessly for so many years evidently lacked the stamina which I must have had to survive the shock of my suddenly arrested flight through space. That the very delusion which drove me to a death-loving desperation should so suddenly vanish would seem to indicate that many a suicide might be averted if the person contemplating it could find the proper assistance when such a crisis impends.

It was squarely in front of the dining-room window that I fell, and those at dinner were, of course, startled. It took them a second or two to realize what had happened. Then my younger brother rushed out, and with others carried me into the house. Naturally that dinner was permanently interrupted. A mattress was placed on the floor of the dining room and I on that, suffering intensely. I said little, but what I said was significant. "I thought I had epilepsy!" was my first remark; and several times I said, "I wish it was over!" For I believed that my death was only a question of hours. To the doctors, who soon arrived, I said, "My back is broken!"—raising myself slightly, however, as I said so.

An ambulance was summoned and I was placed in it. Because of the nature of my injuries it had to proceed slowly. The trip of a mile and a half seemed interminable, but finally I arrived at Grace Hospital and was placed in a room which soon became a chamber of torture. It was on the second floor; and the first object to engage my attention and stir my imagination was a man who appeared outside my window and placed in position several heavy iron bars. These were, it seems, thought necessary for my protection, but at that time no such idea occurred to me. My mind was in a delusional state, ready and eager to seize upon any external stimulus as a pretext for its wild inventions, and that barred window started a terrible strain of delusions which persisted for seven hundred and ninety-eight days. During that period my mind imprisoned both mind and body in a dungeon than which none was ever more secure.

Hospitalization

Knowing that those who attempt suicide are usually placed under arrest, I believed myself under legal restraint. I imagined that at any moment I might be taken to court to face some charge lodged against me by the local police. Every act of those about me seemed to be a part of what, in police parlance, is commonly called the "Third Degree." The hot poultices placed upon my feet and ankles threw me into a profuse perspiration, and my very active association of mad ideas convinced me that I was being "sweated"—another police term which I had often seen in the newspapers. I inferred that this third-degree sweating process was being inflicted in order to extort some kind of a confession, though what my captors wished me to confess I could not for my life imagine. As I was really in a state of delirium, with high fever, I had an insatiable thirst. The only liquids given me were hot saline solutions. Though there was good reason for administering these, I believed they were designed for no other purpose than to increase my sufferings, as part of the same inquisitorial process. But had a confession been due, I could hardly have made it, for that part of my brain which controls the power of speech was seriously affected, and was soon to be further disabled by my ungovernable thoughts. Only an occasional word did I utter.

Certain hallucinations of hearing, or "false voices," added to my torture. Within my range of hearing, but beyond the reach of my understanding, there was a hellish vocal hum. Now and then I would recognize the subdued voice of a friend;

now and then I would hear the voices of some I believed were not friends. All these referred to me and uttered what I could not clearly distinguish, but knew must be imprecations. Ghostly rappings on the walls and ceilings of my room punctuated unintelligible mumblings of invisible persecutors.

A Governor Speaks on Behalf of the Disabled

Franklin D. Roosevelt

On July 13, 1929, then governor of New York Franklin D. Roosevelt made the following speech after completing a tour of his state's hospitals and schools. In his speech, Governor Roosevelt recognizes the advances made by medical science in the treatment of mental illness and other disabilities. But he also calls upon members of Congress to do more to get the mentally and physically disabled the help they need to become active members of society. Finally, FDR urges the public to educate itself about the facilities that exist to help the disabled and the possibilities that exist for cures. As Roosevelt saw it, many more people could be helped if the ignorance and stigma surrounding mental illness and other disabilities was corrected.

Roosevelt's speech drew upon his personal experience. In 1921 at the age of thirty-nine, he contracted polio and lost the use of his legs. Faced with the prospect of being an invalid for the rest of his life, Roosevelt met his disability with a resolve to overcome it. With the help of family and close aides, Roosevelt pursued a political career that led him from the state house to the presidency. During his presidency, FDR's belief that the federal government should take an active role in correcting the ills of society set the stage for the creation of social welfare policy that impacted mental health policy.

At the end of a week's trip across the State of New York inspecting State hospitals and schools, it is natural that my thoughts have run to the tremendous strides made by mankind in health and in education during the past generation.

Franklin D. Roosevelt, "Franklin D. Roosevelt Library, Speech #334, Master Speech File, Franklin D. Roosevelt Papers as President," July 13, 1929. http://www.disability museum.org/lib/docs/2148card.htm.

Take some comparisons. It is less than fifty years ago in this State, and an even shorter time in some other States, that the care of the insane was definitely recognized as a responsibility of the State itself. Many older people can remember the day when mentally deranged members of families were kept at home in seclusion, or else locked up in some local institution which treated the unfortunate victim as a prisoner and not as a patient.

Today, because of an awakened public responsibility and because of great strides in medical science, mental derangement is treated in modern, well-equipped, state-conducted institutions as an illness from which a growing number of patients may and do recover. It is a fact that the percentage of cures is increasing year by year.

Useful Citizens

Take then the class of cases which falls under the head of mental deficiency, and not insanity. It is only a few years ago that the backward child, the boy or girl who did not seem "normal," was classed as an imbecile or an idiot and practically laid to one side by the family in the community. Today the State recognizes the obligation of turning the backward child into a useful citizen, able to take his or her part in life, and modern science proves that this end can be accomplished in the great majority of cases.

Take next the boys and girls who are broadly classed as juvenile delinquents. A generation ago these children were given either sharp physical punishment in their own localities and turned adrift usually to repeat their petty crime and misdemeanors, or else were thrown into a common jail and forced to associate with hardened criminals. Today, Government recognizes its responsibility to the juvenile offender, and the fact that in the large majority of cases these boys and girls can be made law-abiding, hard-working citizens. Again the records show that the millions of dollars expended by the State in this great cause are well invested, and that potential criminals are, in large numbers, being turned into law-abiding citizens.

Medical science and a new public conscience are also obtaining magnificent results in the field of physical, as opposed to mental, disabilities. At one of the institutes for the deaf the other day I spoke of the deaf and dumb. The superintendent corrected me immediately, saying:

"There are very few deaf and dumb people in the world. They are deaf and, as a consequence, have not been able to speak, but they are not dumb."

The instruction of these deaf people is working wonders. Girls and boys are being taught to read lips and to make themselves understood sufficiently to make their own way in the world. It is an interesting fact that there is ready employment for all graduates of our deaf schools.

Salvaging the Disabled

Next we come to the problems of the cripples. A generation ago the crippled had no chance. Today, through the fine strides of modern medical science, the great majority of crippled children are enabled, even though the process may take years, to get about and, in many cases, find complete or practically complete cures. In other words that large part of humanity which used to be pushed to one side or discarded is now salvaged and enabled to play its own part in the life of the community.

This sketch of the development of a generation brings one naturally to the question. What can be done to take further steps in the generation to come? The answer is a simple one. Further progress must of necessity depend on a deeper understanding on the part of every man and woman in the United States. Knowledge of the splendid results already accomplished is not widespread. You can go into thousands of farming districts in this State and you can go into thousands of closely populated wards in our great cities and find ignorance not only of what has been accomplished but of how to go about utilizing the facilities which we already have. There are literally hundreds of thousands of cases of boys and girls in the United States hidden away on the farm or in the city tenements, boys and girls who are mentally deficient or crippled or deaf or blind. Their parents would give anything in the world to have their mental or physical deficiencies cured, but their parents do not know how to go about it.

Educating the Public

In other words, education as to simple facts is of vital importance in every State of the Union, and this education is necessary not only for the dwellers on the remote farms and in the crowded tenements, but it is equally necessary for millions of people who now consider themselves well educated.

I wonder, for example, just how many members of the legislatures in the forty-eight States, just how many members of the Congress of the United States know what is being done by their own State Governments or by the Federal Government in taking care of the mentally or physically crippled. I wonder how many of them have taken steps in their own home districts to bring forward those who need care and are now not getting that care.

I wonder how many so-called leading citizens in any town in the United States know what facilities are offered by State and private institutions, or know what great possibilities for cure exist today with the development of modern medical science.

In other words, the progress which will be made in the coming generation will depend not only on the development and extension of governmental activities and of medical discoveries, but just as important, on the education of the already so-called educated people in this development. Through their efforts thousands of children will receive benefits of modern science which they would otherwise not receive.

This is a problem that demands a crusade. The progress of the past fifty years has been great, but we have marched only a short way. The extension of the work must go on until every child in the United States can be assured of the best that science, government assistance and private aid can give.

It is a task that appeals to our humanity, but it is a task that appeals also to our future economic success. Every citizen, man, woman or child, who is unable to take his or her part in the normal life of modern civilization is a drag on our economic life. Good humanity and good economics demand that the work must go on.

Calling for the Reform of the State Asylum

Albert Deutsch

The nation's first mental asylums were constructed from the 1830s through the 1850s by various states. At the time, some were considered exemplary institutions for the humane care and cure of the mentally ill. Following the model established by Thomas Kirkbride at the Pennsylvania Hospital for the Insane in Philadelphia, these "Kirkbride" mental asylums were spacious, well-maintained, and well-staffed facilities where treatment stressed orderliness, gentle but firm routines, and rest. Within this environment, doctors believed they could cure their patients. Asylums were easily beset by a host of problems, however. Overcrowding was one of the most serious as the number of patients in asylums grew. For example, in 1890 New York State had 13,434 institutionalized patients. In 1910, that number had increased to 31,280. During the Great Depression of the 1930s, the situation worsened as funds for the deteriorating institutions disappeared and state hospitals became custodians of the indigent poor and elderly.

The downward slide continued into the 1940s when Albert Deutsch (1905–1961), an investigative journalist and self-taught historian of the mentally ill published an exposé on the conditions in the nation's state mental asylums. An excerpt from his book, The Shame of the States, *follows. In it, he describes conditions in Manhattan State Hospital.*

Back in 1887 the intrepid girl reporter, Nellie Bly, whose name is now legendary in the newspaper world, feigned insanity and had herself committed to the New York City Lunatic Asylum on Ward's Island in the East River. Nellie emerged with a red-hot exposé series entitled, "Ten Days in a Madhouse." Her articles, which appeared in Joseph Pulitzer's *New York World*, dealt largely with sensational charges that sane people were being railroaded to "lunatic asylums" by scheming relatives in cahoots with crooked lawyers and alienists [psychiatrists]. Nellie cited the case with which she had faked her way into one as an example of how simple it was to dupe the asylum doctors.

The asylum-railroading theme, popular in Nellie Bly's time as a horror-story vehicle, has worn threadbare. Cases of malicious railroading of sane people to mental hospitals are of rare occurrence. Ample safeguards have been built up against the practice.

Nonetheless, as you walk through the wards of the institution exposed by Nellie Bly—taken over by the State of New York a half-century ago and now known as Manhattan State Hospital—you see many cases that don't properly belong there. More than half of the 4,000 patients on Ward's Island are "seniles"—elderly folk whose mental processes have deteriorated because of arteriosclerosis (hardening of the arteries) or other conditions due to old age. Many of these have developed the harmless eccentricities often seen in old people—querulousness, memory gaps, childish traits, etc. Their families, finding them troublesome burdens, dump them in state hospitals in lieu of sending them to the poorhouse. They are shipped to mental hospitals mainly because there is a terrible lack of decent homes for the aged at rates the average family can afford to pay. Then, too, it is far more difficult to keep a feeble old father or mother in a cramped city apartment than on a farm where there's plenty of room.

"We've got to take them," Dr. Frederick MacCurdy, State Mental Hygiene Commissioner, told me. "But it would seem that more suitable institutional provision should be made for this group—perhaps in hospitals for the chronically ill."

The piling up of these "crotchety" old people in our mental institutions, people who can't be helped by psychiatric treatment, is one of the gravest problems of our state hospital system. They tie up psychiatric personnel and facilities that are desperately needed to treat actively the acute and hopeful cases of mental disorder.

They jam the wards of the Manhattan State Hospital, where they are sent in large numbers because of the institution's proximity to the center of the metropolis. About 60 per cent of Manhattan's patients are over sixty years of age; some are past ninety. That's why Manhattan State has such a terrific mortality rate; about one out of six patients dies in the course of a year.

An Aged and Decaying Hospital

The institution itself is aged and decaying. Some of its buildings date back to the Civil War period. In 1923 its tinder-box buildings were swept by a horrible fire in which 21 patients and employees lost their lives. As a result of this holocaust, the state floated a $50,000,000 bond issue to finance a statewide hospital construction and fireproofing program.

But by 1933 the institution had become so hopelessly unfit that it was officially condemned. Its total abandonment no later than 1943 was ordered by legislative enactment. The pressure of chronic overcrowding on other state hospitals, added to the war crisis, caused a postponement in the abandonment plan till 1948. Now the state plans gradually to rebuild the hospital instead of giving it up entirely. A 3,000-bed institution is proposed, to occupy fifty acres on Ward's Island in place of the one hundred and fifty acres now covered. The rest of the Island will be turned back to New York City to be used as a park and recreational center.

The present institution is in an appalling state of deterioration and disrepair as a result of the years of neglect in expectation of abandonment. It is grossly overcrowded and undermanned, like most state hospitals. Some of its wards are crowded double beyond capacity.

A survey of Manhattan State Hospital was made in 1942 by Dr. Samuel W. Hamilton, leading mental hospital expert and past president of the American Psychiatric Association, with the assistance of Miss Mary E. Corcoran, R.N. They noted, in their confidential report to the mental hygiene authorities, a deterioration of staff morale at the hospital in addition to physical deterioration.

Low Morale and Overwork

"An unhappy frame of mind has prevailed in the organization during the last several years," they reported, "while disintegration of the hospital had been agreed on and appeared inevitable. Conservatism, always a strong force in an old institution, was strengthened so that it has been sometimes difficult to persuade the whole organization of the need or even the propriety of steps in advance. What has 'always been done' seemed the only right standard. It is not easy to restore an active aggressive spirit to an organization that for several years has been permeated with a genteel gloom."

This low level of staff morale was evident in several Manhattan State Hospital doctors I talked to. The hospital has some fine psychiatrists on its staff—men who were attracted to it because of its convenient location. It has had a long tradition of active medical treatment, going back to the time when Dr. Adolf Meyer, the great American psychiatrist, made his headquarters there.

Manhattan State is still an active treatment center, in comparison with other state hospitals. Its tradition is maintained largely by the frequent contacts with men from the various medical schools and hospital centers of New York who use it as a research and teaching institution.

But staff doctors can't practice good psychiatry when they have to handle hundreds of patients apiece. One had a load of more than 800 patients, spread over three different buildings, including many on suicidal and homicidal wards.

The average doctor at Manhattan State Hospital, I was told, spends about half his time in paper work—checking patients in and out, making up requisition orders in triplicate and quadruplicate, counting clothes, bed sheets, towels, writing up case reports, accident reports, death certificates, etc. On Sundays only one physician was left in charge of a total of 2,500 patients spread over 32 wards. Besides the impossible task of making rounds on all these wards, the Sunday physician had to see visitors and attend to necessary paper work.

"It means that the doctor is exhausted, the patient is neglected, and the family is discouraged," one physician observed. . . .

Manhattan State Hospital receives mainly two types of mental patients—the very feeble and the very disturbed—both of whom can be transported long distances only with great difficulty or danger.

Both the physically feeble and the mentally disturbed patients are in need of special attention, which makes the problem of undermanning more serious at Manhattan than at other institutions. Nearly one fourth the regular ward jobs were unfilled at the time of my official visit, and 106 of the 432 ward attendants and nurses on the payroll were away on passes, vacations, or sick leave. I was much impressed, however, by the good caliber of a number of hard-working, sympathetic ward nurses and attendants.

Shortage of trained personnel was one reason for the relatively high accident rate among patients of Manhattan State. An official monthly report listed at least 12 serious accidents among patients during April, 1946, four of which terminated in death. Here are some samples:

Fracture neck of right femur. Caused by fall—pushed by another patient. Resulted in death.

Fracture of nose. Caused by altercation with another patient.

Fracture of left hip. Accidental fall here. Patient died.

Fracture right hip. Accidental fall here.

At Manhattan, as at most state mental hospitals, there is a form of labor exploitation that needs long-overdue correction. A considerable number of able-bodied patients are put at institutional labor on a full eight-hours-a-day basis—in the coal yards, laundry, repair shops, etc. But they get no pay for their full-time work. They get only extra rations of tobacco. Time was, at Manhattan, when patient-workers were paid ten dollars a month as recompense. This payment, niggardly enough, was canceled some years ago. It is a good policy to give patient-workers some monetary returns for their labor. It gives them a sense of independence, of being able to earn something. It helps build up self-confidence so strikingly lacking in many mental patients. It's a pity that the old policy was scrapped.

Exploitation and Neglect

I have seen patients even more miserably exploited in other state hospitals. I've seen them, in some places, reduced to slaves and serfs, worked for 12 and 14 hours a day, seven days a week, with no return but candy and tobacco handouts. Sometimes this exploitation operates under the guise of "industrial therapy," when the real motive is not to speed the patient's recovery but to squeeze all possible labor out of him.

Shortly before the day of my official, announced visit to Manhattan State Hospital, I made a preliminary, unannounced inspection of some of the wards. I found several in indescribable stages of filth and general neglect, especially on the women's side.

But when I was officially shown around by Superintendent Travis, these same wards were meticulously scrubbed and tidied up. Wards teeming with untended patients had almost miraculously been emptied, and one which had on my earlier visit presented a bedlamic scene was now transformed into one of patient-less quiet and order.

It was quite evident that Dr. Travis possessed a noble consideration for the sensitivity of visitors to his institution and was bent on avoiding as much unpleasantness as possible. As one institutional employee later told me: "Gee, you must be something special. We sure did some tall cleaning up for you."

It must be said, in fairness, that Dr. Travis and his staff are doing everything possible to keep the decaying, doomed institution as clean as circumstances permit. It's mighty hard, with plaster falling constantly in some wards, paint peeling off the walls in huge blobs, and floors rotting steadily. The location of the hospital in the middle of the East River makes the job of warding off river rats a most difficult one.

An old-timer told me: "We're actually better off than we were a while ago in the way of keeping down rats and vermin, in spite of present appearances. You should have been here a few years ago, when one poor family came to claim a dead relative in the morgue. When the light was turned on, there was a big rat right on the chest of the corpse."

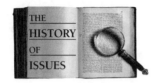

CHAPTER 3

Revolutionary Changes Lead to the Modern Mental Health-Care System

Chapter Preface

The post–World War II era was marked by dramatic changes in the history of mental health in the United States. The institutionalization of the mentally ill in asylums (later called state hospitals) fell out of favor as more psychiatrists left the much-criticized state hospitals to work in private practice and in community clinics. The federal government and its organization, the National Institute of Mental Health (NIMH), which wanted to see funding for mental health care transferred from the old state hospitals to community-based clinics, supported their transition. The impact of this changeover was profound: Before 1948, more than half of all states had no mental health-care clinics; one year later, all but five states had one or more. By the mid-1950s, the United States had about twelve hundred psychiatric clinics. The numbers of community-based psychiatric clinics continued to grow in the following decades.

New treatments such as electroconvulsive therapy, psychosurgery (in the form of lobotomy), and the use of psychoactive drugs (such as lithium and Thorazine) also contributed to the change in the nation's mental health-care system. These therapies appealed to many doctors because they enabled them to better manage patients' depression or schizophrenia. The new therapies not only held out hope of a cure for the chronically ill but also presented a solution to the problem of hospital overcrowding. Both the medical establishment and the public responded with enthusiasm for what they perceived to be groundbreaking science. In theory they approved of the mainstreaming of patients back into the community and the shuttering of the old state hospitals. Opponents of psychiatry, civil rights advocates for the mentally ill and social reformers who decried the idea of insane asylums also added their support to deinstitutionalization.

Unfortunately, the safety net of community psychiatric clinic combined with outpatient care that was supposed to provide comprehensive services for the mentally ill did not materialize the way the federal and state governments and the NIMH had envisioned. Too many of the mentally ill persons released from state hospitals during the 1960s, 1970s, and 1980s had no homes to go to, no families to support them, and were unable to live independently. Within the municipalities that were supposed to absorb them (and were largely unprepared for their role), the mentally ill found themselves unable to afford basic housing, dependent on drugs and alcohol, or incapable of managing their prescribed medications. The unkempt man or woman ranting on the city subway or roaming the countryside with all their belongings stuffed into a few bags became a source of concern to the public and an indelible symbol of the failure of the mental health-care system in the late twentieth century.

The following chapter outlines the developments in mental health treatments and philosophy that developed into the deinstitutionalization movement. It then examines the progress of that movement, which succeeded in reducing the population of mental hospitals while creating, in the view of many critics, a host of new problems.

The National Institute of Mental Health Is Established

National Institute of Mental Health

In 1946 President Harry S. Truman signed into law the National Mental Health Act to support research into the causes of mental illness, to train health professionals, and to award grants to states to help them set up clinics and mental health-care treatment centers. The act led to the creation in 1949 of the National Institute of Mental Health (NIMH) to direct the nation's mental health policy. NIMH later became part of the National Institutes of Health, a component of the Department of Health and Human Services.

At first NIMH had a goal of providing a vision for the future rather than a specific agenda. In the words of first director Robert Felix, NIMH's mental health policy was designed "to make mental health a part of the community's total health program." The leaders of the early NIMH made mental health services available—via community clinics—to emotionally disturbed children, adults able to live outside a hospital setting, and persons in the early stages of mental illness. Since its founding nearly sixty years ago, NIMH has broadened its scope to include behavioral and social science research in all areas of mental health. These include drug addiction, eating disorders, and suicide prevention. NIMH is also a major disseminator of information on all aspects of mental health. It publishes statistics on the number of mentally ill people in the United States, provides the latest news on investigations into the causes of mental illness, prints resource materials for specialists and laypersons, and directs the public to organizations that provide mental health ser-

National Institute of Mental Health, "NIH Almanac—Organization: National Institute of Mental Health," July 20, 2006. www.nih.gov/about/almanac/organization/NIMH.htm#history National Institutes of Health.

vices. An excerpt from the 2006 mission statement of NIMH and a chronology of events in its history is included in the following selection.

The mission of the National Institute of Mental Health (NIMH) is to reduce the burden of mental illness and behavioral disorders through research on mind, brain, and behavior.

In the United States, mental disorders collectively account for more than 15 percent of the overall "burden of disease"—a term that encompasses both premature death and disability associated with mental illness. Mental disorders occur across the life span, from very young childhood into old age.

Investments made over the past 50 years in basic brain and behavioral science have positioned NIMH to exploit recent advances in neuroscience, molecular genetics, behavioral science and brain imaging; to translate new knowledge about fundamental processes into researchable clinical questions; and to initiate innovative clinical trials of new pharmacological and psychosocial interventions, with emphasis on testing their effectiveness in the diagnostically complex, diverse group of patients typically encountered in frontline service delivery systems. NIMH-funded investigators also seek new ways to translate results from basic behavioral science into research relevant to public health, including the epidemiology of mental disorders, prevention and early intervention research, and mental health service research.

Diverse scientific disciplines contribute to the design and evaluation of treatments and treatment delivery strategies that are relevant and responsive to the needs of persons with and at risk for mental illness. A thrust of this research is to eliminate the effects of disparities in the availability of and access to high quality mental health services. These disparities, which impinge on the mental health status of all Americans, are felt in particular by many members of ethnic/cultural, minority groups, and by women, children, and elderly people.

In this era of opportunity, NIMH is strongly committed to scientific programs to educate and train future mental health researchers, including scientists trained in molecular science, cognitive and affective neuroscience, and other disciplines urgently needed in studies of mental illness and the brain.

Mechanisms of Support. The NIMH provides leadership at a national level for research on brain, behavior, and mental illness.

Funding Researchers and Educating the Public

Under a rigorous and highly competitive process, the institute funds research project and research center grant awards and contracts to individual investigators in fields related to its areas of interest and to public and private institutions. NIMH also maintains and conducts a diversified program of intramural and collaborative research in its own laboratories and clinical research units at the National Institutes of Health [NIH].

NIMH's informational and educational activities include the dissemination of information and education materials on mental illness to health professionals and the public; professional associations; international, national, state, and local officials; and voluntary organizations working in the areas of mental health and mental illness.

A Chronology of Key Events: 1940s–1960s

1946—On July 3 President Truman signs the National Mental Health Act, which called for the establishment of a National Institute of Mental Health. The first meeting of the National Advisory Mental Health Council (NAMHC) was held on August 15. Because no federal funds had yet been appropriated for the new institute, the Greentree Foundation financed the meeting.

1947—On July 1 the PHS [Public Health Service] Division of Mental Hygiene awarded the first mental health research grant (MH-1) entitled "Basic Nature of the Learning Process" to Dr. Winthrop N. Kellogg of Indiana University.

1949—On April 15 the NIMH was formally established; it was one of the first four NIH institutes.

1955—The Mental Health Study Act of 1955 (P.L. 84-182) called for "an objective, thorough, nationwide analysis and re-evaluation of the human and economic problems of mental health." The resulting Joint Commission on Mental Illness and Health issued a report, *Action for Mental Health* that was researched and published under the sponsorship of 36 organizations making up the Commission.

1961—*Action for Mental Health*, a 10-volume series, assessed mental health conditions and resources throughout the United States "to arrive at a national program that would approach adequacy in meeting the individual needs of the mentally ill people of America." Transmitted to Congress on December 31, 1960, the report commanded the attention of President John F. Kennedy, who established a cabinet level interagency committee to examine the recommendations and determine an appropriate federal response.

1963—President Kennedy submitted a special message to Congress—the first Presidential message to Congress on mental health issues. Energized by the President's focus, Congress quickly passed the Mental Retardation Facilities and Community Mental Health Centers Construction Act (P.L. 88-164), beginning a new era in Federal support for mental health services. NIMH assumed responsibility for monitoring the Nation's community mental health centers (CMHC) programs.

1965—During the mid-1960s, NIMH launched an extensive attack on special mental health problems. Part of this was a response to President [Lyndon B.] Johnson's pledge to apply scientific research to social problems. The Institute established centers for research on schizophrenia, child and family mental health, suicide, as well as crime and delinquency, minority group mental health problems, urban problems, and later, rape, aging, and technical assistance to victims of natural disasters. A provision in the Social Security Amendments of 1965 (P.L. 89-97) provided funds and a framework for a new Joint Commission on the Mental Health of Children to recommend national action for child mental health. . . .

Alcohol abuse and alcoholism did not receive full recognition as a major public health problem until the mid-1960s, when the National Center for Prevention and Control of Alcoholism was established as part of NIMH; a research program on drug abuse was inaugurated within NIMH with the establishment of the Center for Studies of Narcotic and Drug Abuse. . . .

1970s–1990s

1970—Dr. Julius Axelrod, an NIMH researcher, won the Nobel Prize in Physiology or Medicine for research into the chemistry of nerve transmission for "discoveries concerning the humoral transmitters in the nerve terminals and the mechanisms for their storage, release and inactivation." He found an enzyme that terminated the action of the nerve transmitter noradrenaline in the synapse and which also served as a critical target of many antidepressant drugs.

In a major development that reaped untold benefits for people suffering from manic-depressive illness (bipolar disorder), the FDA [Food and Drug Administration] approved the use of lithium as a treatment for mania, based upon NIMH research. The treatment led to sharp drops in inpatient days and suicides among people with this serious mental illness and to immense savings in the economic costs associated with bipolar disorder.

Also during this year, the Comprehensive Alcohol Abuse and Alcoholism Prevention, Treatment, and Rehabilitation Act (P.L. 91-616) established the National Institute of Alcohol Abuse and Alcoholism within NIMH.

1972—The Drug Abuse Office and Treatment Act established a National Institute on Drug Abuse within NIMH. . . .

1975—The community mental health centers program was given added impetus with the passage of the CMHC amendments of 1975.

1977—President [Jimmy] Carter established the President's Commission on Mental Health on February 17 by Executive Order No. 11973. The commission was charged to review the mental health needs of the Nation, and to make recommendations to the President as to how best to meet these needs. First Lady Rosalyn Carter served as the Honorary Chair of the commission. . . .

1980—The Mental Health Systems Act—based on recommendations of the President's Commission on Mental Health and designed to provide improved services for persons with mental disorders—was passed. NIMH also participated in development of the National Plan for the Chronically Mentally Ill, a sweeping effort to improve services and fine-tune various Federal entitlement programs for those with severe, persistent mental disorders.

1981—President Ronald Reagan signed the Omnibus Budget Reconciliation Act of 1981. This act repealed the Mental Health Systems Act and consolidated ADAMHA's [Alcohol, Drug Abuse, and Mental Health Administration's] treatment and rehabilitation service programs into a single block grant that enabled each State to administer its allocated funds. With the repeal of the community mental health legislation and the establishment of block grants, the Federal role in services to the mentally ill became one of providing technical assistance to increase the capacity of State and local providers of mental health services. . . .

Dr. Roger Sperry, a longtime NIMH research grantee, received the Nobel Prize in Medicine or Physiology for discoveries regarding the functional specialization of the cerebral hemispheres, or the "left" and "right" brain. . . .

1992—Congress passed the ADAMHA Reorganization Act (P.L. 102-321), abolishing ADAMHA. The research components of NIAAA [National Institute on Alcohol Abuse and Alcoholism], NIDA [National Institute on Drug Abuse] and NIMH rejoined NIH, while the services components of each institute became part of a new PHS agency, the Substance Abuse and Mental Health Services Administration (SAMHSA). The return to NIH and the loss of services functions to SAMHSA necessitated a realignment of the NIMH extramural program administrative organization. New offices are created for research on Prevention, Special Populations, Rural Mental Health and AIDS.

1993—NIMH established the Silvio O. Conte Centers program to provide a unifying research framework for collaborations to pursue newly formed hypotheses of brain-behavior relationships in mental illness through innovative research designs and state-of-the-art technologies.

NIMH established the Human Brain Project to develop, through cutting-edge imaging, computer, and network technologies, a comprehensive neuroscience database accessible via an international computer network. . . .

1996—NIMH, with the NAMHC [National Advisory Mental Health Council], initiated systematic reviews of a number of areas of its research portfolio, including the genetics of mental disorders; epidemiology and services for child and adolescent populations; prevention research; clinical treatment and services research. At the request of the NIMH director, the NAMH Council established programmatic groups in each of these areas. NIMH continued to implement recommendations issued by these Workgroups. . . .

1999—U.S. Surgeon General David Satcher released *The Surgeon General's Call To Action To Prevent Suicide*, in July, and the first *Surgeon General's Report on Mental Health*, in December. NIMH, along with other Federal agencies, collaborated in the preparation of both of these landmark reports.

In the late 1990s, NIMH began to strengthen its efforts to include the public in its priority setting and strategic planning processes, instituting a variety of approaches in which to insure increased public participation.

The NIMH expanded and revitalized its public education and prevention information dissemination programs, including information on suicide, eating disorders, and panic disorder, in addition to the ongoing Institute educational program, Depression: Awareness, Recognition, and Treatment (D/ART).

NIMH also launched an initiative to educate people about anxiety disorders, to decrease stigma and trivialization of these disorders, and to encourage people to seek treatment promptly.

NIMH included members of the public on its scientific review committees reviewing grant applications in the clinical and services research areas. . . .

Early 2000s

2000—NIMH launched a 5-year communications initiative in March 2000 called the Constituency Outreach and Education Program, enlisting nationwide partnerships with state organizations to disseminate science-based mental health information to the public and health professionals, and increase access to effective treatments.

NIMH co-hosted two town meetings in Chicago on the mental health needs of minority youth and related research. The first meeting, held in April 2000, focused on behavioral, emotional, and cognitive disorders; the impact of violence; the criminalization of youth with treatment needs; service system issues; barriers to treatment; and barriers to research. The July 2000 meeting addressed the prevention of sexually transmitted diseases, such as HIV, and the role of the family and society in stemming the spread of HIV, as well as the increase in violence. Members of the general public, parents, teachers, school officials, guidance counselors, and professionals in the health, family assistance, social services, and juvenile justice fields attended the meetings. . . .

2001—NIMH launched several long-term, large-scale, multi-site, community-based clinical studies to determine the effectiveness of treatment for bipolar disorder (also called manic-depressive illness); depression in adolescents; antipsychotic medications in the treatment of schizophrenia, and management of psychotic symptoms and behavioral problems associated with Alzheimer's disease; and subsequent treatment alternatives to relieve depression. . . .

2002—NIMH published a national conference report entitled "Mental Health and Mass Violence: Evidence-Based Early Psychological Intervention for Victims/Survivors of Mass Violence: A Workshop to Reach Consensus on Best Practices." While most people recover from a traumatic event in a resilient fashion, the report indicates that early psychological intervention guided by qualified mental health caregivers can reduce the harmful psychological and emotional effects of exposure to mass violence in survivors. NIMH and the Department of Defense, along with other Federal Agencies and the Red Cross collaborated in the preparation of this report. . . .

2003—Real Men. Real Depression campaign launched to raise awareness about depression in men and create an understanding of the signs, symptoms and treatment options available. The campaign is designed to inspire other men to seek help after hearing from real men talking about their experiences with depression, treatment and recovery.

Psychoactive Drugs and Their Role in the Treatment of the Severely Mentally Ill

David Healy

The introduction of powerful psychoactive drugs in the treat-
ment of the severely mentally ill changed the scenario of mental
health care in the United States, according to psychiatrist and
writer David Healy. The discovery of chlorpromazine in 1952 by
researchers at the French pharmaceutical company Rhône-
Poulenc and its subsequent use with patients suffering from
schizophrenia and other disabling mental disorders was greeted
by the medical establishment and the public as one of the great-
est triumphs in modern medicine. Patients who had previously
been categorized as hopelessly manic or delusional responded to
the new drug (marketed in the United States under the name
Thorazine) in amazing ways. As described by Healy, the use of
Thorazine and other drugs such as lithium and reserpine al-
lowed patients to be released from overcrowded state asylums,
made skeptical psychiatrists open to the use of pharmaceuticals
in their practices, and placed drug companies in the forefront of
the treatment of the mentally ill.

Chlorpromazine [did] not sedat[e] patients in the usual way. Sedatives usually put patients into a sleep from which they could be roused only with difficulty, and when they did wake up they would be groggy or drowsy. But patients on chlorpromazine although apparently asleep, responded rapidly to any approach, knew immediately where they were, and were able to react quickly. It was as though they had retreated from the outside world but could reengage if needed.

David Healy, *The Creation of Psychopharmacology*, Cambridge, MA: Harvard University Press, 2002, pp. 91, 96–100. Copyright © 2002 by the President and Fellows of Harvard College. All rights reserved. Reprinted by permission of the publisher.

A number of patients appeared to wake up. [One researcher] details the case of Phillippe Burg, a man who had been sunk in an inaccessible psychotic state for several years before the advent of chlorpromazine. No treatment had helped him. Everything had been tried but nothing worked. Over several weeks of treatment, he began to emerge from his torpor and communicate. Thereafter he progressed so rapidly that the staff allowed him to go out with his mother. They went to dinner at a famous haunt of Ernest Hemingway's, Closerie des Lilas.

A typical example of how chlorpromazine helped psychosis is the case of a barber from Lyon who had been hospitalized for several years with a chronic psychosis and was unresponsive to his environment. When given chlorpromazine, he awoke from this stuporous state and told his doctor, Jean Perrin, that he now knew where he was and who he was, and that he wanted to go home and back to work. Perrin responded by challenging him to give him a shave. The open razor, water, and towels were produced and the patient set about doing his job perfectly. Either Perrin had considerable nerve or the transformations were truly extraordinary.

In Bassens Hospital, Pierre Lambert was faced with a patient who had been psychotic for years, frozen in a series of postures. No one knew anything about him. He responded as dramatically as Perrin's barber to chlorpromazine, in one day. He greeted Lambert and the nursing staff on the ward round, asking them for some billiards balls, which he proceeded to juggle. . . .

Thorazine

Chlorpromazine was slow to come to American psychiatry. . . . SK&F [American pharmaceutical company Smith, Kline & French] had only a limited interest in hospital psychiatry, where another drug, reserpine, was already making inroads. In the United States, office practice was where the money was to be made. Would the new drug, marketed as Thorazine, compete with the amphetamines or barbiturates or SK&F's own Dexamyl? In fact, had SK&F waited a few more months it might have given up on chlorpromazine because of the advent of another drug that swept the market in office psychiatry in 1956: Miltown.

But in 1953, SK&F asked several U.S. psychiatrists to test the new drug, and some agreed to do so. William Winkelman in Philadelphia used it in office practice to treat nervous conditions, concluding that Thorazine was helpful but not free of side effects. Frank Ayd also used it in office practice and found that the new drug caused dystonias, jaundice, and a range of other problems. Vernon Kinross-Wright in Houston undertook a study and reported significant benefits, but he was treating hospitalized patients.

A twist of fate shaped developments. Chlorpromazine was sold by Rhône-Poulenc in Canada. . . . One day Heinz Lehmann, a German-Canadian who worked at the Verdun Hospital, read about chlorpromazine while taking a bath. The next day, he ordered supplies of the drug. He recruited a resident to help and gave chlorpromazine to seventy patients. He also gave it to some nurses to study how it worked. Many of the nurses suffered a severe drop in blood pressure but the patients began to respond. Astonished, Lehmann saw the awakening that psychiatrists in Paris, Lyon, and Basel had witnessed. As he later put it, if these patients or their relatives had been told that the price of these recoveries would be death in two years, they would have taken the two years of restored life. These were unexpected transformations in patients who had previously had no prospect of recovery.

Lehmann raced to publish his results, worried that he might be scooped by someone in the United States. His efforts led to his sharing the 1957 Lasker Prize, . . . [and] he became a powerful advocate for chlorpromazine. . . .

Hospitals Eager to Use the Drug

In the meantime, SK&F contacted Henry Brill at Pilgrim State Hospital in New York. As the commissioner for mental health in New York state, Brill was a key figure, and he all but instructed several of his colleagues to try out the new drug. Later he convened a meeting of New York State psychiatrists. . . . A range of asylum and office practitioners, . . . who came to hear about the new drug heard many reports of its benefits. The SK&F representatives at the meeting were besieged with requests for samples.

State mental hospital doctors were so eager to use the drug that when chlorpromazine was finally launched as Thorazine, in 1955, even though the license application had been for an antiemetic [a drug that prevents vomiting], the take-up in psychiatry was astonishing—SK&F reportedly took in $75 million the first year the drug was sold. To understand this figure, it needs to be appreciated that some of the American state asylums, such as Pilgrim State in New York, had up to 15,000 residents. Everyone got the new drug. Al Kurland, an early psychopharmacologist, was so impressed with the effects that he mortgaged his house to buy shares in SK&F.

Like their counterparts in Europe, psychiatrists quickly realized that a new kind of psychiatry was needed, one with outpatient clinics to monitor the functioning of patients newly released from asylums. American psychiatrists quickly increased the dose of chlorpromazine much more than the Europeans had done, . . . giving 2 grams of chlorpromazine per day and reporting if not benefits for every patient, then at least a lack of toxicity. . . .

A New Drug for Office Practice

In the United States, SK&F was faced with a challenge that did not develop elsewhere. The 1955 meeting of the American Psychiatric Association (APA) should have been dominated by Thorazine. But while Thorazine was on stage, the whispers in the wings were of an even newer drug, Miltown (meprobamate), which was launched in the second half of 1955. This was a drug for office practice. Only 20 percent of the membership of the APA were hospital psychiatrists at the time. No other Western country had this distribution of psychiatric power. By any reckoning, therefore, while Miltown might never have made a splash elsewhere, Thorazine's time at center stage in American psychiatry should have been short. The fact that it survived the inroads of Miltown and remained at the center of the scientific stage is compelling testimony to the recognition that chlorpromazine truly was a different drug.

Miltown's popularity did have one long-lasting influence on Thorazine. It made it into a major "tranquilizer." The term *tranquilizer* had first been used in 1953 by F. F. Yonkman, an employee of the Ciba pharmaceutical company, to describe another drug, reserpine. But the term had still not achieved currency, when Miltown's creator, Frank Berger, used it to keep people from thinking of his new drug as a sedative, like the barbiturates. The idea of sedation was not compatible with a treatment that would allow people to get on with their lives, so Miltown became a tranquilizer. And since Thorazine's profile overlapped that of reserpine, it too became known as a tranquilizer. But Thorazine and Miltown differed so much in their profiles of action that a distinction was very quickly established between the major tranquilizers, such as chlorpromazine and reserpine, and the minor tranquilizers, such as Miltown and later Librium and Valium. Most American practitioners did not consider Thorazine an antipsychotic until many years later. Meanwhile in Europe, chlorpromazine was on its way to becoming regarded as a neuroleptic. Not until the 1900s did practitioners worldwide come to regard both the major tranquilizers and the neuroleptics as antipsychotics.

Studying the Drugs

The distinctive American contribution to the story of chlorpromazine was the effort to evaluate the new technologies. Confronted with the dominance of psychoanalysts within American psychiatry, the proponents of the new pharmacotherapies felt the need to justify use of drugs to a greater extent than did psychiatrists elsewhere. Accordingly, the Psychopharmacology Research Center was established within the National Institute of Mental Health (NIMH). Ralph Gerard and Jonathan Cole, the director of the new center, convened a meeting in September 1956 to look into means of evaluating the new agents. Shortly thereafter, a series of studies was conducted that demonstrated beyond reasonable doubt that the new drugs had measurable effects. This discovery of evaluative technologies . . . has done at least as much as the discovery of the new drugs to shape the modern era in psychiatry.

From State Mental Hospital to Psychiatric Center

George W. Dowdall

State mental hospitals have played a key role in caring for the seriously mentally ill since the early years of the nation. Created by reformers, doctors, and concerned government leaders, they were envisioned to be places of humane treatment for the chronically ill. Over time, however, they became overcrowded, physically rundown, and insufficiently funded. The derisive term "snake pit" (after a famous novel of the 1940s about a patient in a state asylum) was applied to these institutions. In the 1960s, 1970s, and 1980s states began to close some of their asylums and release patients into the community in a process known as deinstitutionalization. Care for this population was shifted to mental health centers. The state asylums that remained open, such as Buffalo State Hospital in New York, gradually transformed themselves from being custodians of the ill into a provider of various services. This ongoing transformation—which involved, among other things, the use of new drugs and the shifting of patients to nursing homes and group homes—is the subject of the following selection by sociologist George W. Dowdall.

How was one reasonably representative state hospital transformed into a contemporary public psychiatric center? Perhaps because of the stigma still associated with the seriously mentally ill (or even more precisely, with those treated in public hospitals), there has been little written about this transformation, and so this account tries to present a detailed portrait of change, drawn mostly from the hospital's Annual Reports. . . . Most writing on public mental health ignores the

George W. Dowdall, from *The Eclipse of the State Mental Hospital*. Albany: State University of New York Press, 1996, pp. 139–146, 148–149. Copyright © 1996 State University of New York. All rights reserved. Reproduced by permission of the State University of New York Press.

state hospital or gives the impression that little has changed (except perhaps overall size) since deinstitutionalization began in the 1960s; in fact, as the following account makes clear, it is actually the case that little has remained the same at state hospitals since the 1960s, and that such organizations were transformed through a combination of external pressure and internal development, often involving great conflict and tension. The result was a different organizational form. . . .

Deinstitutionalization Begins

Organizational turning points rarely can be fixed with certainty, but the mid-1950s marks the beginning of fundamental change in the character of the Buffalo State Hospital. In New York, an important policy shift began in 1954 with passage of the Community Mental Health Services Act which encouraged the development of local mental health services outside the immense state hospital system. . . .

But the most dramatic change came in psychiatry itself that year. Very soon after their first appearance on the market, new psychoactive drugs were used in several New York state hospitals, including Buffalo:

> The new drugs, chlorpromazine [known in the USA under the brand name Thorazine] and reserpine, were available in trial quantities during the early part of the fiscal year and a very small number of cases were treated up to the time these were reported at the conference on drugs at Creedmoor State Hospital in December 1954. Following this, the drugs were administered to a larger number of patients, and they were first made part of the official monthly report in January 1955. In the remaining three months of the fiscal year, 177 patients received chlorpromazine and 167 received reserpine. Following this, the use of these drugs was markedly increased and evaluation will be made in the next annual report. It may be said, at this time, however, that the use of the new drugs is encouraging. It has not been found that they can entirely replace conventional shock therapies,

but the use of shock therapy has diminished with the expansion of the drug program and a number of people who failed to improve with electric shock and insulin therapy showed gratifying improvement with the new drugs.

Appearing at a time when morale and staff performance seemed to be rising for other reasons, the drugs' introduction into clinical practice helped to strengthen the feeling that major improvements in care were possible. Older therapies (including a few lobotomies) continued, however, and newer approaches such as psychology were expanded modestly. Full-time Catholic and Protestant chaplains and a part-time "Hebrew" chaplain began work, with "a profound effect upon the hospital, its patients and its community relationship." Another 39 staff positions were added, chiefly in ward service, bringing the total to 881 employees. The medical staff was allocated 23 positions, with 20 actually filled. Certified capacity increased to 2,503, but the hospital had on its books 1131 more patients, making overcrowding 41 percent overall. . . .

Changes in Inpatient Care

The 1959 Annual Report contains items that show the increasingly contradictory character of the organization: in some ways a traditional custodial hospital, in other ways an increasingly dynamic institution adapting innovations from the national movement toward community psychiatry. Aided by a transfer of patients to Marcy State Hospital, the decline in patient census continued. But perhaps more significant for the hospital's character was an important change in the character of inpatient care. Patients with grounds privileges increased to 800, with more "open wards" replacing the traditional locked ward. Among the changes was the first year of activity of the Department of Volunteers and an outpatient clinic at the convalescent hospital for Erie County. Outside accreditors gave only conditional and partial approvals, which were due to "overcrowding and the inadequate physical facilities," despite the fact that new laundry, storehouse and bakery buildings had been opened. Perhaps most significant of all were changes in the plans for a new patient building; originally intended for 940, the building was now stripped back to 520 beds; no longer mentioned was the planned 150-bed addition to the reception building. While building plans were cut back, the medical staff was increased from 24 to 29 by the end of the fiscal year, and overcrowding decreased to 32 percent.

The next year saw several other signs of a shifting philosophy of care. Patients with grounds privileges increased from 800 to 1500. The psychiatric staff ran a series of conferences on admission, diagnosis, and release, "intensifying the training program and bringing more clearly into focus the needs of the individual patient." The treatment effort was "advancing consistently with the application of improved methodology.". . .

In 1965, the transformation from custodial to active treatment continued, though again at a pace that must have frustrated those looking for more rapid reform. Overcrowding was reduced to 9.4 percent. A new 100-bed intensive treatment unit opened to rehabilitate patients hospitalized continuously more than two years.

During the late 1960s, major changes took place in both the hospital's physical plant and the character of care. On Oct 21, 1965, Governor Nelson Rockefeller dedicated the new 544-bed Reception and Intensive Treatment Building (named the Strozzi Building, after a former board member). This almost eliminated overcrowding, now down to only 3.4 percent. A number of attendants were trained in the remotivation of long-stay patients, while an experiment had 58 patients working at a canning factory for three months at minimum wage. . . .

New Standards for Patients

But perhaps the most significant change of the entire decade occurred during 1968, when a new statewide policy to control admissions of elderly patients began to change operations at the institution. A "Geriatric Screening Team" became operational in August, 1968. This team, made up of a psychiatrist, a social worker and a community mental health nurse, began to screen all patients age 65 and over, resulting in a significant decrease in the number of elderly patients admitted. Readers of the annual report would not learn that this represented a major savings by the state; those elderly formerly admitted to care at full state expense would now be diverted to nursing homes, where the costs of care would be paid for by federal dollars. . . .

The institution known as the Buffalo State Hospital since 1890 was renamed, in 1974, the "Buffalo Psychiatric Center" (BPC), with the other New York state hospitals also changing their names during this year. New York's Commissioner of Mental Health claimed this change reflected the many new functions that these institutions now performed, beyond the traditional ones of custody and care. In this case, the name change stemmed not merely from organizational public relations, even if one of the consequences of the change was to lessen the connection with a stigmatized past. New York was one of the very few states that attempted to transform its old state hospitals into centers for non-inpatient treatment, so in a real sense the name accurately reflected a profound change in function. It also most certainly reflected the extraordinarily negative image that "state hospital" conjured up in both professional and lay circles.

The Role of Community Mental Health Centers

David Hartley, Donna C. Bird, David Lambert, and John Coffin

In 1963 Congress created Community Mental Health Centers (Cmhcs) to serve all members of the community without re- gard to an individual's ability to pay. In many parts of the coun- try, especially in rural areas, the centers became mental health safety nets for chronically mentally ill people who had been deinstitutionalized—released from mental asylums into the com- munity—but who continued to need treatment. The psycholo- gists and social workers who authored the following paper exam- ine community mental health centers in Maine, Minnesota, and Oregon and each state's funding of its mental health centers. As part of their study, the authors trace the evolving role of CMHCs from the 1960s, with a focus on how presidents, factions within the mental health-care system, and local, state, and federal gov- ernments created an intricate, often helter-skelter way of provid- ing services to a needy population.

The national movement to provide community-based men- tal health services to a broad segment of the U.S. popula- tion began at a 1953 conference on mental health cosponsored by the American Medical Association (AMA) and the Ameri- can Psychiatric Association (APA). Out of this conference came a recommendation for a study to develop national stan- dards for treatment of the mentally ill. In 1955, the World Health Organization published a study indicating the need for community-based treatment of the mentally ill. Several Euro- pean countries were ahead of the U.S. in their development of community-based residential care and outpatient services for

David Hartley, Donna C. Bird, David Lambert, and John Coffin, "The Role of Commu- nity Mental Health Centers as Rural Safety Net Providers, Working Paper #30," Maine Rural Health Research Center, November 2002. Reproduced by permission.

persons with mental illness. In this climate of concern, Congress agreed to sponsor the study recommended by the AMA/APA conference, passing the Mental Health Study Act (PL 84-182) on July 28, 1955.

The study was conducted by a nonprofit corporation, the Joint Commission on Mental Illness and Health, which had been formed by the AMA and APA with partial financing from a major pharmaceutical manufacturer. In 1960, at about the time John F. Kennedy assumed office as President of the United States, the Joint Commission released its report, *Action for Mental Health*. The report recommended building on the structure already developed by state governments using the NIMH [National Institute of Mental Health]-funded community clinic model. This approach was intended to bolster the state hospital system and maintain state control over the clinics.

Deciding Against the States as Providers of Care

The *Action for Mental Health* findings influenced an address President Kennedy made before Congress on February 5, 1963. In this address, Kennedy emphasized poverty as a causal factor in mental illness and called for community prevention efforts specifically directed toward low-income people. Kennedy also proposed a 50-percent reduction in state hospital populations across the country over the next ten years. In response to the report, President Kennedy also formed an interagency task force on mental health headed by his Secretary of Health, Education and Welfare, Anthony Celebrezze. The task force included representatives from the Veterans Administration, Department of Labor, Bureau of the Budget and the Council of Economic Advisors. Professionals from NIMH staffed the group.

The Celebrezze Task Force released its findings in December 1962, proposing a federal categorical grant program that would create a national network of community mental health centers [CMHC]. During the subsequent hearings regarding the proposed Community Mental Health Centers Act, both the Kennedy Administration and Congress elected to follow the Task Force recommendations rather than those from the *Action for Mental Health* study. The moral values of the era, asserting the primacy of civil and human rights, coupled with intensely negative criticism of state governments as providers of care, influenced these choices.

Two Camps and Barriers to Coordination

During the period prior to the adoption of the CMHC Act, members of the psychiatric profession were divided into two camps regarding the preferred model for organizing and delivering mental health services. One supported the health model of mental illness, which focused on prevention, education and community care. The tenets of so-called community psychiatry had much in common with the emerging anti-poverty movement, so these groups tended toward a natural alliance. The other camp took a more traditional, "medical model" stance that focused on expansion of the state hospital system and state government control of community-based services. While the second group, in combination with the AMA, influenced the development of the Joint Commission report, the first group influenced the Celebrezze Task Force and the Kennedy Administration.

Likening community care to "socialized medicine," the AMA also allied itself with state government administrators in opposition to the CMHC Act. The latter vigorously opposed the Act due to the proposed shift in the locus of control and funding away from states. In their defense, most state government leaders supported deinstitutionalization for both humanitarian reasons and as means of controlling rising institutional care costs. Supporters of the public health model blamed state governments for the failings of the institutional mental health system and its well-publicized abuse and neglect of psychiatric patients. The alliance of community psychiatrists and community mental health activists successfully characterized state government leaders as personally responsible for the persistent evils of custodial care. The lingering resentment of state mental health program directors toward the psychiatrists who ran many of the new CMHCs established a persistent barrier to coordination between the two sectors of the public mental health system.

CMHC: From State to Federal Government

President Kennedy signed the Mental Retardation Facilities and Community Mental Health Centers Construction Act (PL 88-164)—commonly known as the CMHC Act—into law on October 31, 1963. It represented a deliberate shift of control over the community mental health system from the states to the federal government. More critically, the Act created a split in authority and responsibility between the state hospital system of institutional care and the system of community-based mental health care intended to serve as a means of controlling admissions to the state hospital system. Over the next 15 years, the census of state and county mental hospitals declined by about two-thirds, while federal funds supported the establishment of more than 500 community mental health centers. In testimony presented to Congress in 1980, NIMH staff reported that 37 percent of the CMHCs served rural areas.

Due to the push to pass comprehensive social legislation in a volatile political climate, the CMHC role described in the Act was broad and open to interpretation. To be illegible for federal funds, centers had to provide the following:

- *Inpatient services*, either directly or through referral by screening patients for hospitalization;

- *Outpatient services*, although neither target populations nor specific services were defined;

- *Partial hospitalization services*, the precursor to day treatment programs for discharged hospital patients;

- *24-hour emergency services*, available as part of at least one of the other three services; and

- *Consultation and education services*, for professionals and community agencies.

The law also encouraged provision of an additional five services (*rehabilitation, diagnosis, pre- and aftercare, research/evaluation* and *training*), which entitled a CMHC to use the "comprehensive" designation. In part because the Act failed to define priority service populations, many CMHCs did not assume responsibility for the aftercare of patients discharged from the state hospitals. While the population of these facilities dropped rapidly during the 1960s in accordance with the goals of the Kennedy Administration and many state legislatures, many people with serious and persistent mental illness were discharged into community settings with little or no follow-up care.

Although the CMHC Act required centers to serve a defined geographic catchment area, the law also included minimal requirements regarding services to low-income people, suggesting merely that centers provide ". . . a reasonable volume of services to the indigent." This is surprising given the deliberate linking of mental illness to poverty expressed by both the Kennedy Administration and the community mental health movement. This lack of specificity regarding the CMHC role in serving low-income populations allowed for considerable latitude in CMHC policies and practices. Provisions of services to low-income people varied significantly from center to center, depending on the extent to which center leadership viewed such activity as mission-critical.

The Issue of Funding

With the expectation that the facilities would eventually become self-sufficient, Congress built time-limited and declining federal support into the CMHC Act. In addition, the initial grants supported construction but not staffing. As a consequence, operating funds were an issue from the inception of the program. Many CMHCs developed serious financial difficulties within a few years of opening. This dilemma prompted them to market services to individuals covered by health insurance at the expense of other, more needy, populations. Some critics argued that the centers under-performed in serving both low-income people and people with serious and persistent mental illness. A more charitable view is that CMHCs were simply overwhelmed with the demands for service and the range of needs of the diverse groups that compromised the very loose definition of those with mental illness and could not respond adequately given their considerable resource limitations. . . .

Community-based mental health services expanded throughout the 1960s and 1970s, in part as a consequence of the growing number of clinicians setting up private practices. Nevertheless, the lack of community-based services for people with serious mental illness coming out of state hospitals remained an apparently intractable problem. Its urgency was amplified in many states by highly publicized class action suits and resulting consent decrees that required state mental health agencies to assume responsibility for redressing the consequences of years of neglect.

In response to these and other concerns, in 1977, President [Jimmy] Carter appointed a Commission on Mental Health to study the need for further changes in the nation's mental health system. The Commission's recommendations, released in 1978, focused on increased funding of mental health services, particularly for people with serious and persistent mental illness and other priority population groups. These recommendations were codified in the Mental Health Systems Act (PL 96-398), which President Carter signed into law on

October 8, 1980, a month before he lost the [presidential] election to Ronald Reagan.

States Are Made Responsible, Again

Ronald Reagan won the 1980 election with promises to reduce government waste and regulation and to return responsibility for many social programs to the states. This platform was known as the New Federalism. One of the keystones of the New Federalism was the Omnibus Budget Reconciliation Act of 1981 (PL 97-35, also known as OBRA 1981). OBRA 1981 and its resulting administrative rules included several provisions directly affecting the status, mission and viability of CMHCs, such as:

- Repealing the Mental Health Systems Act;

- Withdrawing direct federal categorical grant support from the CMHCs and replacing that funding with Alcohol, Drug Abuse and Mental Health Block Grants to the states;

- Through the block grant mechanism, returning to the states the primary authority for deciding how and to whom mental health services should be provided;

- Reducing overall federal funding for mental health service delivery and reallocating funds to substance abuse treatment services;

- Eliminating the federal requirements regarding CMHC utilization reporting; and

- Ceasing to make official use of the term "community mental health center" to describe a unique entity.

Finding Ways to Survive

Both the CMHCs and the state mental health agencies were compelled to adapt to these dramatic changes in the policy and funding environment. . . . The states were already under considerable pressure to move people with serious and persistent mental illness out of state institutions and into the community. Many states took advantage of the shift in control mandated by OBRA 1981 to contract with CMHCs to provide services to de-institutionalized or other priority populations.

With federal support for community mental health services declining by over 20 percent from 1981 to 1983, fears of financial insolvency resurfaced among CMHCs. However, very few CMHCs closed or merged as a result of these changes. As of 1991, 672 (88.3 percent) of the 761 CMHCs in operation in 1981 were still providing services. Reductions in staff and increased efforts to shift services toward paying clientele were common strategies adopted by centers in an effort to assure survival.

By the early 1990s, the picture was starting to get brighter. From 1987 to 1997, state spending on mental health services increased by over 2 percent. Federal spending during the same period increased by over 6 percent, in large part as a consequence of increased reliance on Medicaid funding for these services. The Alcohol, Drug Abuse and Mental Health Administration Reorganization Act of 1992 (PL 102-321) established a community mental health services block grant specifically aimed at supporting services for children with serious emotional disturbances and adults with serious and persistent mental illness.

Who Pays?

While many CMHCs have survived, their service priorities and the locus of control over these priorities have changed substantially. A common practice among CMHCs and other health care providers has been to use revenues produced by paying patients combined with support from federal, state and local government to cover the costs of caring for low income uninsured people. However, a number of forces have combined to change the practices of insurers, providers and government agencies, leaving each less willing to pick up a share of the costs of these so-called safety net populations. . . .

Community mental health centers remain the only real option for mental health treatment for low income uninsured people, yet the availability of services for this population has steadily decreased in the last twenty years. These individuals often sit on CMHC waiting lists for extended periods or are turned away due to a lack of funds for services other than those targeted to priority populations. While Medicaid provides financial access to mental health services for people poor enough to qualify, CMHCs still are caught between state priorities and local need with limited staff and resources.

The Rationale
Behind Deinstitutionalization

Ann B. Johnson

Deinstitutionalization—the process of releasing mental patients from hospitals back into the community—remains controversial to this day. Doctors working in the hospitals, social workers interacting with former patients in mental health-care clinics, and government leaders have different perspectives on the issue and a variety of outlooks on the topic. Ann Braden Johnson, a clinical social worker, criticizes deinstitutionalization for what it failed to deliver: a coordinated system of services that would enable the chronically mentally ill to manage their lives within the community. In Johnson's view, the failure rests in the fact that deinstitutionalization was not planned; rather, it was a grand experiment concocted by the overly optimistic who believed that drugs could cure the mentally ill and that communities could deal with former patients living in their midst. Johnson also implicates psychiatrists who, in her view, abandoned treating chronically ill patients in the hospitals for treating patients with more successful prognoses in community health centers.

The idea that deinstitutionalization was a piece of deliberate social planning seems so rational and so obvious as to go without saying, to people both in and out of the mental health field. It's not true. Deinstitutionalization, which did not even have a name when it happened, was the product of only dimly related forces: the "can-do" postwar American mood, which was one of optimism, faith in the future, and enthusiasm for scientific breakthroughs; the latest in the long line of shocking exposés of heinous conditions in state mental hospitals, which appeared in the late 1940s and the early 1950s; the

Ann B. Johnson, from *Out of Bedlam: The Truth About Deinstitutionalization*, New York: Basic Books, 1990, pp. 24–32, 35–37. Copyright © 1990 by Basic Books, Inc. Reprinted by permission of Basic Books, a member of Perseus Books, L.L.C.

organized activity of the states, which had recognized that the costs to them of lifetime care for the chronically mentally ill were prohibitive; and the profession of psychiatry, which was caught up in a longstanding conflict about the chronic mental illnesses and how best to deal with them. What we now call deinstitutionalization did take place—but it was not planned; it simply happened.

The Nation's Mood in the 1940s

After the Second World War, itself a great triumph for the United States, the country was in a mood to make a radical change in the way it dealt with its chronically mentally ill. This occurred partly because postwar America was a prodigiously optimistic place, and partly because medical science in those years was unusually powerful and popular, thanks in no small measure to its successful campaign against polio in the mid-fifties. Deeply feared, even though it was by no means the most prevalent nor the deadliest disease of the day, polio was a most effective cause for the March of Dimes and other organizations devoted to raising money for medical research. When the Salk [polio] vaccine was made available in 1955, the public was wildly enthusiastic and passionately grateful to medical research. "The magic of science and money had worked. And if polio could be prevented, Americans had reason to think that cancer and heart disease and mental illness could be stopped, too."

At the same time, the public's conscience about its hospitalized mentally ill underwent one of its periodic shakeups, this time because of a national newspaper scandal concerning the traditional neglect of hospitalized mental patients. The conscientious objectors had formed their organization, the National Mental Health Foundation (NMHF), and their demands for hospital reform had attracted no less a spokesman than Albert Deutsch, a journalist whose articles in *PM* [a New York daily newspaper] about the terrible conditions in American mental hospitals were published in 1948 as a widely read book, *The Shame of the States*. An effectively gruesome novel called *The Snake Pit* was published in 1946, whose author, Mary Jane Ward, was said to have been a nurse in a state hospital; if anything, the book's effectiveness and popularity were surpassed when a movie [version] starring Olivia de Havilland appeared two years later. Additional studies of chronic mental illness and institutional care from this period included ones by Lucy Freeman (*Fight Against Fears*) and Mike Gorman (*Every Other Bed*); clearly, the topic was timely and the issue ubiquitous.

What we now call deinstitutionalization came out of the postwar period. One central factor spurred efforts to reduce the state hospital population: State officials could read a spread sheet, and they knew that their continued single-handed support of the huge state hospital patient population would ensure their own bankruptcy. In 1949, the forty-eight state governments took the step—unusual for them—of coming together to discuss what to do about one specific problem, the chronically mentally ill.

The Problem of the States

In preparation for their meeting, officials in each state conducted surveys to establish the baseline condition of their state's hospitals and to determine future needs. All the states reported severe overcrowding of hospitals; a desperate need for modern equipment and facilities, as well as for trained personnel; a preponderance of special-problem patients such as alcoholics and the elderly; a need for preventive treatment; outmoded laws and terminology that tended to emphasize custodial care rather than active treatment; an overuse of involuntary commitment; admissions and discharges based on legal, rather than clinical, considerations; and far too many hospitalized patients who could be discharged if only there were community-based alternatives. . . .

The [state] governors held [a] conference in February 1954, in Michigan, with all the states represented except Arizona and Nevada. At once, the tone was set by G. Mennen Williams of Michigan, who called for a cooperative effort by all the states to reverse the trend of rising hospital population and costs by promoting prevention, early diagnosis, and shorter hospital stays. Dr. Henry Brill, Assistant Commissioner of the New York State Department of Mental Hygiene, forecast a 250 percent increase in the patient population between 1930 and 1965 unless trends changed. A recurrent theme reported from the conference was the charge that states spent too much money on hospital construction and not enough on research that would render those hospitals obsolete. For the first time, the state leaders pledged to pool their experiences with administration, personnel recruitment, and research; one contemporary observer was particularly impressed by the representatives' eagerness to sponsor research that might eventually restore mentally ill citizens to normal life rather than to devise ever more elaborate structures for locking them up. . . .

Although the governors' activities were impressive and their recommendations novel, the council's proceedings cannot be described as a formal planning meeting at which the future of the state hospitals was decided in an organized and thoughtful way, complete with the thorough design of alternative systems of care for the patients then in the states' mental hospitals. Theirs was a first step—and a tentative one at that. For movement on a larger political scale, the federal government had to be involved; and for professional authority and endorsement, the mental health establishment—which is to say, organized psychiatry—had to be included.

The NIMH Plays a Role

Much of the political activity of organized psychiatry at that time took place under the aegis of the National Institute of Mental Health (NIMH), which in those years was expanding

141

at an amazing rate: from its initial appropriation of $870,000 in 1950, its budget grew to $18 million in 1956 and to $68 million in 1960, all of it, unlike the money that supported the chronic patients, in federal dollars. From the beginning, the NIMH, which was to set the course for the mental health field for years to come, did not have as its focus either the public mental hospitals or the severely mentally ill. Its first director, Robert Felix, wrote off the chronically mentally ill by calling for "an attack on mental illness [that] must reach beyond the more serious hospitalized cases to those persons in the community with psychoneuroses and character and behavior disorders that cause untold suffering and economic loss." Thus, one of the most prestigious professional organizations in the field of mental health openly turned away from the chronically mentally ill and the institutions charged with their care; instead, the NIMH favored patient populations that could be expected to prove more rewarding to practitioners. Ironically, the initiative originally undertaken by the states to address the needs of the hospitalized mentally ill in a new way by expanding the scope of psychiatry to the community had become the occasion for their abandonment by mainstream psychiatry.

Giving Up on the State Hospitals

Five years later, the president of the American Psychiatric Association (APA), Harry C. Solomon, made his organization's intention to give up on the state hospitals and their problems equally clear in his presidential address to the organization's national conference: "I do not see how any reasonably objective view of our mental hospitals today can fail to conclude that they are bankrupt beyond remedy. I believe therefore that our large mental hospitals should be liquidated as rapidly as can be done in an orderly and progressive fashion." Citing Massachusetts' diminishing state hospital patient census as an example, he observed that "the first signs of self-liquidation are already evident. . . . This suggests that if the trend continues, less bed space will be required." Less callous and indifferent to the needs of the already diagnosed than his counterpart at the NIMH, Solomon was nonetheless startlingly woolly-headed and vague as he outlined his amorphous plans to relocate the state hospital caseload in general hospital psychiatric wards, new clinics, day hospitals, night hospitals, private mental institutions, rehabilitation or after-care programs, and new facilities for the elderly—all of which he cheerfully, if naively, believed to be extant. Similarly, he made enthusiastic plans for psychiatrists in private practice to take on the chronically mentally ill, declaring them to be "equipped for and interested in" the population—an amazing and unbelievable statement for which he offered no documentation. Next, he mentioned a proposal he admitted was sketchy and incomplete to resettle the long-term chronic patients in "a colony or home rather than in a hospital," with rehabilitation as the central service and a multidisciplinary staff. Admitting that he had no idea how to implement his plan, he nevertheless made an admirably honest assessment of the state of the art in his day: "One must face the fact that we are doing little by way of definite treatment of a large number of our chronic hospital population. It is not even the case that we are providing them with first class environmental care, much less loving and tender care."...

The planned shift to community-based care was a radical notion: move a nonexistent service to an untried market. The assumption underlying the shift was that the chronically mentally ill would be accommodated in hypothetical new clinics along with the mildly troubled, but no one knew just how this would work, since it had never been tried. It is possible that everyone involved, from the NIMH and the APA on down, firmly intended to ensure that the new clinics would treat the seriously ill; but it seems extremely unlikely that the truly deranged were much on the minds of those thrilled with the prospect of a glorious new day of significant medical advances in the treatment of the mentally ill in the community.

The Federal Government Gets Involved

The federal government got involved in the mental health issue when the combined pressures of the nation's governors, the NIMH, the APA, public health organizations, and various citizens' groups prompted them to undertake a full-scale study of the mental health needs of the country. . . . The federal study was cosponsored by senators John F. Kennedy and Lister Hill and was initially known as the Mental Health Study Act of 1955 (PL 84-182). The act appropriated $1,250,000 for research into the diagnosis and treatment of mental illness and established the Joint Commission on Mental Illness and Health. The joint commission, under its director, Jack Ewalt, spent five years in deliberation and study, issuing its final report, *Action for Mental Health*, in 1961. . . .

The commission recommended huge outlays of federal funds to abolish the state hospital system as then constituted in favor of community-based treatment facilities coordinated with the old hospitals in smaller form, with additional funds for research and professional training.

As it happens, the process of emptying the state hospitals had been under way for over five years by the time the joint commission's report came out; in fact, the event was taking place even as it was under examination and debate by the commission in its effort to plan for mental health's future—so much for strategic planning and long-range thinking. In retrospect, this placement of the cart before the horse seems particularly unfortunate, for among the commission's most salient observations were some it made about the readiness of the general public to accept the mentally ill, whom it had stigmatized and banished for years. . . .

A Debate Within Psychiatry: Who to Treat?

The philosophical debate within academic psychiatry over whether or not to include long-term hospitals in the overall design of the community mental health centers was argued on the highest intellectual plane, which is to say it was made so abstract as to be removed from reality and therefore of questionable usefulness. At the time, practicing psychiatry's most pressing problem was that it had a great many patients stuck away in decrepit old buildings where very little of therapeutic value was going on. To appear to weigh the relative merits of dealing with those patients, on the one hand, or addressing larger issues, such as reaching out to the community to prevent future problems, on the other, seems disingenuous at best and downright dishonest at worst. After all, prevention and planning for psychiatry's future could easily have been begun even as the profession went on dealing with its preexisting problems, so there was no imperative to neglect old tasks in favor of the new. The chronic caseload, needless to say, existed no matter what the profession did. Nevertheless, the pretense of compelling choice was used to justify irresponsibility—not for the first time, and probably not for the last. . . .

In the end, professional psychiatry prevailed over the curious consortium assembled to be the joint commission. The task force sent President Kennedy programmatic recommendations that called for creation of community mental health centers, funds to staff them, funding for states to acquire inventories of existing resources in order to plan for the future, federal support to improve the quality of service in state and county facilities, federal encouragement of insurance companies to cover psychiatric treatment, and the apparently obligatory funds for professional training and research. As ultimately negotiated, the Community Mental Health Center Construction Act of 1963 (PL 88-164) represented a compromise between the hospital-oriented joint commission and the community-oriented task force. . . .

Deinstitutionalization was not planned; it just happened. It would have happened someday in any case, and maybe it would have worked better with a little more advance planning. At certain points in its course, the shift of the chronic population from hospitals to communities proceeded like a juggernaut.

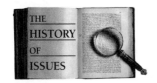

CHAPTER 4

Mental Health Activism

Chapter Preface

The mental health reformers of the nineteenth century clamored for more-humane treatment of the mentally ill and supported the asylum setting as the best method of treatment. That view was discarded during the twentieth century as mental health-care professionals, government leaders, and advocates for the mentally ill called for the reintegration of the mentally ill into society. The resulting mainstreaming of the mentally ill into society during the late twentieth century has forced Americans to deal with issues surrounding the ability of the mentally ill to look after themselves, and to what extent the state should remain responsible for their well-being. Do the rights of the individual to his or her autonomy and personal freedom outweigh the duty of the community to protect all the residents and ensure that the mentally ill will not be left to die on the streets?

This fundamental question is complicated by the fact that the system of community care envisioned by the deinstitutionalization movement has proven faulty, leaving towns and cities across the nation to deal with a new subgroup of citizens: the mentally ill homeless who would not accept treatment or assistance even if their lives were endangered.

Several developments during the late twentieth century illustrate how society grappled with these issues. Some mentally ill patients, acting in concert with dedicated social workers and doctors, acted on their own behalf to provide a solution. They saw the need for a special community within the larger community that would provide a safe place for them to work toward independence. One group—the founders of Fountain House in New York City—developed a widely emulated model of the halfway house/clubhouse for the mentally ill. There, the mentally ill could regain work habits, study, make and meet friends, and manage their daily lives within a supportive community. In time, mental health-care workers and community leaders recognized the important role of halfway houses in helping the mentally ill feel connected to the rest of society.

The government and the courts also tried to address many of the issues concerning the deinstitutionalized mentally ill during this time. Laws were passed to establish greater protection for the mentally ill. In several cases, the courts dealt with important questions: Under what conditions could the state commit an individual to a mental institution without their consent? What constitutes "dangerousness" when deciding whether mentally ill persons pose a threat to themselves or others? Are hospitalized mentally ill patients entitled to a certain standard of care and treatment? The resulting decisions came down strongly in support of the civil rights of the mentally ill. The mentally ill had the right to plead on their behalf, could not be committed without detailed proof, and could decline treatment under specific circumstances. At the same time, different laws and court cases addressed the other extreme: What can government do to prevent the mentally ill from endangering the rest of society?

The following chapter examines the efforts of groups, individuals, federal and state government, and the legal system to answer some of the most difficult questions concerning the responsibility a society has for the care of its mentally ill members.

Regaining One's Personhood: A Personal Account

Jacqueline Peckoff

In 1948 a group of former patients at Rockland State Hospital in New York State started Fountain House, a self-help program located in a New York City mansion. There, men and women recovering from mental illness work, relax, study, socialize, and find their way back into the community. In a setting described as a "clubhouse," members coordinate with a professional staff to create and organize the programs run by Fountain House. Since 1948, Fountain House has served more than sixteen thousand individuals and has provided the model for similar programs in thirty-two countries. The enduring mission of Fountain House is to help men and women with mental illness achieve their goals and be respected as coworkers, neighbors, and friends.

In the following selection, Fountain House member Jacqueline Peckoff describes her experiences leading up to her hospitalization and the life she found at Fountain House in the late 1980s. For Peckoff, her arrival at Fountain House was the beginning of her transformation from patient to person.

Before coming to Fountain House, I had a 21-year work history, with only a few jobs. Each lasted between 6 and 8 years. I always enjoyed working because it gave so much structure and meaning to each day. Weekends, holidays, and vacations were special, and I enjoyed my leisure time. My last job before coming to Fountain House was a supervisor of what was called the order department. This was at a large company that manufactured jeans. This job entailed processing orders that were sent in by retail stores when they needed more

Jacqueline Peckoff, "Presentation to the Fifth International Seminar on the Clubhouse Model, St. Louis, Missouri," Fountain House/*fountainhouse.org*,1989. Reproduced by permission.

jeans. I would figure out how many of each size were needed by looking at previous orders that we had filled for them. This would tell us how many jeans they had sold. I would use a comptometer. For people who were born in the olden days, like myself, that was a sort of computer that was used in those days. I also supervised six other people, people who did similar work.

During this job, I became ill several times and needed to be hospitalized due to severe depression. I was able to return to work as soon as I was discharged from the hospital and it was good to know that they still needed and wanted me. I was very grateful, but often wondered why they were so understanding. I found out when I came to Fountain House. We had a transitional employment slot at this very company.

After working at this company for about four years, I had to be hospitalized once again. This time things were different: I had lost all my confidence and developed a terrible fear of working. For about a year, I was going in and out of the hospital, and then there were no more holidays, weekends, and vacations; every day was the same and no longer had any special meaning. At the end of the year, I was sent to a state hospital, where I was told that not only would I never work again, but that I would spend the rest of my life in a hospital.

Well, that got me real mad, and that was because I knew that in spite of all the shock treatment and heavy medication I had taken, I still had a life to live and needed out.

In a relatively short time, I got better. But to be discharged, you needed a place to live, which I already had, and a discharge plan. I was sick and tired of making elephants out of clay. They said I had a real talent, but little did they know I went to camp when I was 10 years old and that was the only thing I could make. I had already made enough trivets so that not only I, but both my sisters, could each serve ten hot dishes at a time and never have to worry about burning the table. I was sick of groups, and no, I'm not against therapy. I was just tired of having it every day. So, what was I going to do?

As I pondered this, all of a sudden, I remembered that during one of my hospitalizations, I had met a woman that I shall never forget; who said she was a member at a place called Fountain House. I couldn't remember anything that she told me, except you could return to work if you went there. So, I told the doctor that I wanted to go to Fountain House. This was arranged, and I went to orientation while I was still in the hospital. When I first came to Fountain House, I was extremely quiet and withdrawn (this is where I usually get a laugh) and sat in a corner in the Clerical Unit for about 4 months.

During this time, I was always looking around and noticed members and staff working on the switchboard, the newspaper, research projects, and attendance. Members and staff would try to encourage me to get involved, and, though I did not at the time, something was going on because I came in mostly every day even though it took me an hour and a half to get there. One day, one of the staff members came over to me and asked me if I would like to go to a tour guide meeting. That was the last thing I wanted to do. But because she had helped me to get financial assistance when I needed it, I said okay. That was almost 14 years ago, and I'm still a tour guide.

Now you know how long I've been a member, but don't worry, I'm not going to take you through all 14 years. I've done many different things at Fountain House during the years: operated the switchboard, worked with my colleagues during their training, worked the copy machine. I could probably go on all day telling you all the things I've done, but I won't. I also worked on several transitional employments (TE's) and did return to independent employment, but became ill again. At one time, I also went to typing school. . . .

When I was on TE, most of the time I also came to Fountain House for the other half of the day. When I was not working full-time or going to school, I would come in as I still do today, for 6 hours or longer. Now I spend so much time at the clubhouse because I am doing real work, and know that I am expected and needed. To be needed, to me, means more to me than anything else in my life, and it also means that I am living a meaningful life. I share many responsibilities with others, and when I don't come in, it's nice to know I'm missed.

From Patienthood to Personhood

Until [a couple of] years ago, I still had a strong need to be a patient, and did many things so that I could be hospitalized. I realize now that this was part of my illness, but I still have a hard time talking about it. I took overdoses and faked heart attacks and appendicitis; I would say I was hearing voices, although I no longer was, just so I could get the attention I thought I needed. All this did was confuse me because I was so convincing that the doctors believed me, and I myself no longer knew what was real and what wasn't.

One evening when I was once more hospitalized and was lying in bed and feeling extremely depressed, I decided that I had to change my ways. The very next day, I told my doctor what I had been doing all these years. That was the beginning of my emergence from patienthood to personhood.

When I returned to Fountain House, I felt awful about what I had done, but was unable to share this with staff members I was close to. During the last year, I have been able to tell my family (actually it was 2 weeks ago that I told them) and some friends. And today, I choose to tell all of you because I know that you'll understand and I can finally let go.

I am now doing more work at Fountain House than I have ever done before. I am a co-manager of a switchboard placement agency at the *Village Voice,* which is a really fun place to work. I still work with colleagues, and for the last year have been on the faculty of the National Clubhouse Expansion Program. I have done many consultations at different clubhouses all around the country. For the last two months, I have worked very hard at helping to get the agenda together for the seminar [at which she delivered this talk]. I also made phone calls to the clubhouses and worked on the computer so that the presenters would know which workshop they were part of. I won't tell you how I pressed the wrong button one day and wiped out the whole program. Now you know why I had to make phone calls and you never got your printouts in advance.

At the very moment I wrote this, a very special friend of mine was in the hospital. She was discharged, so she is home now, but this was the fifth time in a year. I felt that part of the reason is that she has been going to day treatment programs for a long time, where they focus on your illness and not what you can do. They had all kinds of groups to keep you busy, but no real work so that you can feel needed.

This is the first time in six years that I have been out of the hospital for more than a year. I am now getting a great deal of positive attention from other people. I'm the happiest I have ever been in my whole life, and I sincerely believe it's because of the work-ordered day and the opportunities offered to me at the clubhouse.

The U.S. Government Protects the Rights of the Mentally Ill

United States Congress

In 1986 the Protection and Advocacy for Individuals with Mental Illness Act (PAIMI) was enacted. This legislation required the states to establish services for the prevention of the abuse and neglect of individuals with mental illness who were or had recently resided in hospitals. Neglect includes inadequate or inappropriate treatment, nutrition, clothing, health care, and discharge planning. The legislation marked a major event in mental health activism; that is, the move to protect and advocate for the rights of mentally ill adults and children. Each state has a PAIMI protection and advocacy program that includes the investigation of hospitals, nursing homes, and group homes. PAIMI also ensures that the mentally ill have access to support services in the community so they can live as independently as possible. In 2000 Congress expanded PAIMI's mandate to all individuals with mental illness, including people living in the community in all settings.

The following article is taken from the law's restatement of a bill of rights for the mentally ill.

It is the sense of the Congress that, as previously stated in title V of the Mental Health Systems Act, [42 U.S.C. 9501 et seq.] each State should review and revise, if necessary, its laws to ensure that mental health patients receive the protection and services they require, and that in making such review and revision, States should take into account the recommendations of the President's Commission on Mental Health and the following:

United States Congress, "Protection and Advocacy for Individuals with Mental Illness Act, Subchapter II. U.S. Code, sec. 10841," February 27, 2007. frwebgate.access.gpo.gov.

(1) A person admitted to a program or facility for the purpose of receiving mental health services should be accorded the following:

(A) The right to appropriate treatment and related services in a setting and under conditions that—

(i) are the most supportive of such person's personal liberty; and

(ii) restrict such liberty only to the extent necessary consistent with such person's treatment needs, applicable requirements of law, and applicable judicial orders.

Rights

(B) The right to an individualized, written, treatment or service plan (such plan to be developed promptly after admission of such person), the right to treatment based on such plan, the right to periodic review and reassessment of treatment and related service needs, and the right to appropriate revision of such plan, including any revision necessary to provide a description of mental health services that may be needed after such person is discharged from such program or facility.

(C) The right to ongoing participation, in a manner appropriate to such person's capabilities, in the planning of mental health services to be provided such person (including the right to participate in the development and periodic revision of the plan described in subparagraph (B)), and, in connection with such participation, the right to be provided with a reasonable explanation, in terms and language appropriate to such person's condition and ability to understand, of—

(i) such person's general mental condition and, if such program or facility has provided a physical examination, such person's general physical condition;

(ii) the objectives of treatment;

(iii) the nature and significant possible adverse effects of recommended treatments;

(iv) the reasons why a particular treatment is considered appropriate;

(v) the reasons why access to certain visitors may not be appropriate; and

(vi) any appropriate and available alternative treatments, services, and types of providers of mental health services.

(D) The right not to receive a mode or course of treatment, established pursuant to the treatment plan, in the absence of such person's informed, voluntary, written consent to such mode or course of treatment, except treatment—

(i) during an emergency situation if such treatment is pursuant to or documented contemporaneously by the written order of a responsible mental health professional; or

(ii) as permitted under applicable law in the case of a person committed by a court to a treatment program or facility.

(E) The right not to participate in experimentation in the absence of such person's informed, voluntary, written consent, the right to appropriate protections in connection with such participation, including the right to a reasonable explanation of the procedure to be followed, the benefits to be expected, the relative advantages of alternative treatments, and the potential discomforts and risks, and the right and opportunity to revoke such consent.

(F) The right to freedom from restraint or seclusion, other than as a mode or course of treatment or restraint or seclusion during an emergency situation if such restraint or seclusion is pursuant to or documented contemporaneously by the written order of a responsible mental health professional.

(G) The right to a humane treatment environment that affords reasonable protection from harm and appropriate privacy to such person with regard to personal needs.

(H) The right to confidentiality of such person's records.

(I) The right to access, upon request, to such person's mental health care records, except such person may be refused access to—

(i) information in such records provided by a third party under assurance that such information shall remain confidential; and

(ii) specific material in such records if the health professional responsible for the mental health services concerned has made a determination in writing that such access would be detrimental to such person's health, except that such material may be made available to a similarly licensed health professional selected by such person and such health professional may, in the exercise of professional judgment, provide such person with access to any or all parts of such material or otherwise disclose the information contained in such material to such person.

(J) The right, in the case of a person admitted on a residential or inpatient care basis, to converse with others privately, to have convenient and reasonable access to the telephone and mails, and to see visitors during regularly scheduled hours, except that, if a mental health professional treating such person determines that denial of access to a particular visitor is necessary for treatment purposes, such mental health professional may, for a specific, limited, and reasonable period of time, deny such access if such mental health professional has ordered such denial in writing and such order has been incorporated in the treatment plan for such person. An order denying such access should include the reasons for such denial.

(K) The right to be informed promptly at the time of admission and periodically thereafter, in language and terms appropriate to such person's condition and ability to understand, of the rights described in this section.

The Right of Access

(L) The right to assert grievances with respect to infringement of the rights described in this section, including the right to have such grievances considered in a fair, timely, and impartial grievance procedure provided for or by the program or facility.

(M) Notwithstanding subparagraph (J), the right of access to (including the opportunities and facilities for private communication with) any available—

(i) rights protection service within the program or facility;

(ii) rights protection service within the State mental health system designed to be available to such person;

(iii) system established under subchapter I of this chapter to protect and advocate the rights of individuals with mental illness; and

(iv) qualified advocate; for the purpose of receiving assistance to understand, exercise, and protect the rights described in this section and in other provisions of law.

(N) The right to exercise the rights described in this section without reprisal, including reprisal in the form of denial of any appropriate, available treatment.

(O) The right to referral as appropriate to other providers of mental health services upon discharge.

(2)(A) The rights described in this section should be in addition to and not in derogation of any other statutory or constitutional rights.

(B) The rights to confidentiality of and access to records as provided in subparagraphs (H) and (I) of paragraph (1) should remain applicable to records pertaining to a person after such person's discharge from a program or facility.

(3) (A) No otherwise eligible person should be denied admission to a program or facility for mental health services as a reprisal for the exercise of the rights described in this section.

(B) Nothing in this section should—

(i) obligate an individual mental health or health professional to administer treatment contrary to such professional's clinical judgment;

(ii) prevent any program or facility from discharging any person for whom the provision of appropriate treatment, consistent with the clinical judgment of the mental health professional primarily responsible for such person's treatment, is or has become impossible as a result of such person's refusal to consent to such treatment;

(iii) require a program or facility to admit any person who, while admitted on prior occasions to such program or facility, has repeatedly frustrated the purposes of such admissions by withholding consent to proposed treatment; or

(iv) obligate a program or facility to provide treatment services to any person who is admitted to such program or facility solely for diagnostic or evaluative purposes.

(C) In order to assist a person admitted to a program or facility in the exercise or protection of such person's rights, such person's attorney or legal representatives should have reasonable access to—

(i) such person;

(ii) the areas of the program or facility where such person has received treatment, resided, or had access; and

(iii) pursuant to the written authorization of such person, the records and information pertaining to such person's diagnosis, treatment, and related services described in paragraph (1)(I).

(D) Each program and facility should post a notice listing and describing, in language and terms appropriate to the ability of the persons to whom such notice is addressed to understand, the rights described in this section of all persons admitted to such program or facility. Each such notice should conform to the format and content for such notices, and should be posted in all appropriate locations.

The Role of the Court-Appointed Guardian

(4) (A) In the case of a person adjudicated by a court of competent jurisdiction as being incompetent to exercise the right to consent to treatment or experimentation described in subparagraph (D) or (E) of paragraph (1), or the right to confidentiality of or access to records described in subparagraph (H) or (I) of such paragraph, or to provide authorization as described in paragraph (3)(C)(iii), such right may be exercised or such authorization may be provided by the individual appointed by such court as such person's guardian or representative for the purpose of exercising such right or such authorization.

(B) In the case of a person who lacks capacity to exercise the right to consent to treatment or experimentation under subparagraph (D) or (E) of paragraph (1), or the right to confidentiality of or access to records described in subparagraph (H) or (I) of such paragraph, or to provide authorization as described in paragraph (3)(C)(iii), because such person has not attained an age considered sufficiently advanced under State law to permit the exercise of such right or such authorization to be legally binding, such right may be exercised or such authorization may be provided on behalf of such person by a parent or legal guardian of such person.

(C) Notwithstanding subparagraphs (A) and (B), in the case of a person admitted to a program or facility for the purpose of receiving mental health services, no individual employed by or receiving any remuneration from such program or facility should act as such person's guardian or representative.

Revisiting the Case of Alberta Lessard

Dave Umhoefer

In the 1971 case of Alberta Lessard, a diagnosed schizophrenic who was accused of attempted suicide, a Milwaukee court struck down Wisconsin's commitment law as unconstitutional and set a narrow standard as to what constitutes "dangerousness." The court decided that involuntary commitment to a mental institution was only permissible when "there is an extreme likelihood that if the person is not confined he will do immediate harm to himself or others." In addition, the court for the first time required that commitment proceedings provide the mentally ill with all the protections given to a criminal suspect—the right to counsel, the right to remain silent, and a standard of proof beyond a reasonable doubt. Lessard had enlisted Milwaukee Legal Services to gain her release from the hospital she was taken to after she was arrested; legal services then brought a class-action suit on behalf of all adults held on the basis of the state's involuntary civil commitment laws.

The case of Alberta Lessard illuminated the broad and vague scope of commitment laws in the states. Advocates for Lessard and those like her also assumed that commitment seriously damaged the mentally ill person. They proposed that commitment was "a massive curtailment of liberty" and that the mentally ill might be better off foregoing treatment than being hospitalized for treatment. The impact of Lessard's case—which coincided with the deinstitutionalization of the mentally ill—is the topic of the following article, which follows up on the impact of Lessard's case thirty years after the court decision.

Dave Umhoefer, "Teacher's case opened door for mentally ill," *Milwaukee Journal Sentinel*, August 27, 2000. Republished with permission of *Milwaukee Journal Sentinel*, conveyed through Copyright Clearance Center, Inc.

Alberta Lessard, the diminutive former West Allis school-teacher with the squeaky voice, is a most unlikely revolutionary. But it was her case, first brought almost three decades ago, that transformed the nation's mental health laws.

Lessard, diagnosed as a paranoid schizophrenic, was taken into custody by police in October 1971 after what police said was a suicide attempt. She disputed both her diagnosis and the allegation that she was trying to kill herself.

With the help of lawyers from Milwaukee Legal Services, Lessard fought for—and won—constitutional protection for the mentally ill so they could no longer be held against their will without the right to counsel. The case also established their rights to remain silent, to challenge evidence and to a standard of proof beyond a reasonable doubt. (Since then, the law has been modified to a standard of clear and convincing evidence.)

Before Lessard's case, Wisconsin and most other states allowed a person to be detained for as long as 145 days on the petition of anyone claiming to have the person's best interest at heart.

Lessard's case led to the exodus of mental patients from hospitals across the country. In Milwaukee County, the number of beds at the Mental Health Complex, at 9455 Watertown Plank Road in Wauwatosa, dropped from more than 4,000 on any given day to fewer than 300 today [in August 2000].

The Result of Reform

Now, a quarter of a century after the U.S. Supreme Court affirmed [Alberta Lessard's] rights, it is clear the reforms that followed the decision have failed to deliver a better life for hundreds of Milwaukee County's mentally ill. Many of the mentally ill were ushered out of mental hospitals without a decent place to live. Today [in August 2000], hundreds of Milwaukee's mentally ill roam the streets homeless, languish in prison or suffer in nursing homes and other group facilities where they get little, if any, appropriate care.

Homeless shelter workers estimate that half of the 2,000 or so who live on Milwaukee's streets are chronically and persistently mentally ill. Prison and jail officials say one-third of the 2,500 inmates at the county jail and the House of Correction are suffering from a major mental illness. Hundreds more mental patients are being warehoused in nursing homes without adequate care to address their needs, civil rights advocates say.

"They are the new lepers," says Sister Ann Catherine, a nun who works with the mentally ill in Milwaukee. "People want to tuck them into a corner and forget about them."

No one pines for the days of Nurse Ratched of *One Flew Over the Cuckoo's Nest* fame, when a person could be locked up simply for looking strange. Still, thousands of the mentally ill, once hospitalized, now no longer have a clean place to sleep and enough food to eat.

After the Lessard case, the federal government began putting pressure on local governments to empty mental hospitals by requiring an accounting for all those who would be receiving federal funds for care. The idea, says Beverly Malone, deputy to U.S. Surgeon General David Satcher, was to incorporate the mentally ill into the fabric of the community, where they could be much more productive. The problem, she says, is that local governments did not provide adequate housing or jobs programs.

"When we deinstitutionalized in the early 1970s, it was based on a European model that presumed there would be resources in the community to care for the mentally ill," she says. "That hasn't happened."

Innovative programs—some public and others private—treat, safely house and employ some of the mentally ill, but the programs' limited scope leaves many to cope on their own in the outside world. Even less is available for the mentally ill who have alcohol and drug problems, physical disabilities or troubles with the criminal justice system.

The push to deinstitutionalize, accelerated by the Lessard case, has even the fiercest civil libertarians complaining that the county has gone too far in cutting back the in-patient care for the mentally ill.

"Voluntary patients who need, want, and could most benefit from help are turned away every day," says Tom Zander, the lawyer who represented Lessard several times over the years and has passionately maintained that involuntary commitment is wrong. As units of the Milwaukee County Mental Health Complex "are closing down for economic reasons, the facility is becoming simply a detention center for involuntary patients," he said.

Too Great a Change?

Robert Pledl, another lawyer who has defended hundreds of mentally ill clients over the past 20 years, says the pendulum has swung too far, so that the sickest and neediest of the mentally ill are being denied.

"I've handled plenty of cases over the past few years where we let the guy go and he was really darn dangerous. Voluntary treatment is great, but it doesn't work for everybody," he said.

Workers at the Mental Health Complex say they are frustrated by the dwindling number of beds. Four psychiatrists have quit since June [2000], when the county cut another 23-bed long-term care ward. There are 71 long-term beds remaining. Managers there say the resignations were by doctors who left for higher salaries, but they concede that they are troubled by the departures.

The psychiatrists either couldn't be reached or refused to comment.

"I'm very worried, you bet," says Kathleen Eilers, administrator of the county's Mental Health Division. "We don't want to turn this into a place where any Joe with a medical degree can get a job."

Medical staffers say the cutbacks have them concerned.

"We're sending some very sick people back onto the streets," says Cheryl Meyer, a nurse at the Mental Health Complex's emergency room.

Just as alarming, she says, is that patients are being discharged before they are ready, in order to make way for new patients in crisis.

Psychiatrists such as Michael McBride and Vance Baker say they have become increasingly frustrated with the county rejecting patients of theirs who have been in desperate need.

For his part, Jon Gudeman, medical director at the complex, says he, too, is frustrated by the lack of care some mental patients receive. He blames a part of that on Wisconsin law, which does not allow a doctor to initiate an order to detain a mentally ill person. Only a police officer can do that.

Gudeman says the county is hindered, in part, by the very size of the Mental Health Complex. It serves the largest population base of any institution of its kind in the country, he says. The average mental hospital serves a population of 75,000 to 200,000, while the Milwaukee complex serves the entire county, or roughly 1 million people. Gudeman says the county should consider abandoning the centralized care approach and running more, smaller mental health care facilities in the community.

"Maybe it's time for a little rethink," he says. "Maybe it's time to put it all together again."

Lessard, who turned 80 [in August 2000], is not happy with the legacy of her lawsuit. She thinks life has gotten worse, not better, for the mentally ill since her lawsuit began in October 1971. As irony would have it, Lessard has tried occasionally over the years to get help at the Mental Health Complex, only to be turned away.

"They said I wasn't sick enough," she says.

A Writer Looks at Mental Illness in Her Community

Bebe Moore Campbell,

Families with mentally ill members face a myriad of challenges that range from getting their relative into care to accessing social service entitlements such as Medicaid and Social Security Disability. In the following excerpt from a 2005 interview with Los Angeles–based Public Broadcasting Service talk-show host Tavis Smiley, author Bebe Moore Campbell discusses her own experiences taking care of a relative with bipolar disorder and how it inspired her novel, 72 Hour Hold. *Campbell took the title from the amount of time an individual is allowed to be held in a psychiatric facility against his or her will if he or she meets the criteria of posing a danger to self or others. In the interview the author discusses her frustrations with the mental health-care system and her desire to shine a light on African Americans' reluctance to discuss mental illness in their community.*

Bebe Moore Campbell was born in Philadelphia and was a teacher and freelance journalist before she published her first novel, Your Blues A'int Like Mine. *She died in 2006 at the age of fifty-six.*

Tavis: Bebe Moore Campbell is the author of several acclaimed novels including 3 *New York Times* best sellers. She's also a past recipient of the NAACP Image Award for literature. Her latest book is receiving terrific reviews. It's called *72 Hour Hold*, her fifth novel. Bebe, nice to see you.

Bebe Moore Campbell: Nice to see you, too, Tavis.

Tavis: I read—was it the *L.A. Times?* I read somewhere the other day, somebody proclaimed this the summer—I'm paraphrasing here—the summer of the black female novelist?

Bebe Moore Campbell, interviewed by Tavis Smiley, "Bebe Moore Campbell Interview with Tavis Smiley," *www.pbs.org*, September 15, 2005. Reproduced by permission.

Campbell: Well, there's a lot of us. Yeah, I saw the story.

Tavis: There's a lot of y'all. You're out, Terry McMillan is out, Benilde Little is out. Missing a couple of 'em, but there are 5 or 6 of y'all with major books out this summer.

Campbell: Pearl Cleage.

Tavis: Did y'all design that? Did y'all have a conference call one day and say . . .

Campbell: You know we didn't.

Tavis: Ha ha ha! Let's put a book out there, all of us, each of us.

Campbell: Well, it's a good summer. It's a good summer thing to do.

Tavis: Is that a good thing? And I ask is it a good thing because when I see stories like that, on the one hand I would assume that you and all your other sister friend authors want to be judged by their own work. On the other hand, it doesn't hurt when somebody writes a big feature piece and it goes around the country saying that all these books are out this summer. Is that grouping something that offends you?

Campbell: Well, the attention is a big plus. I'm not offended by being in the company of these women because they're stellar and they're good writers and we all write our own stories. So it still is news when a lot of African American women are writing books at the same time. I hope we get to the point where that's not news. But we're not there yet, Tavis.

Tavis: Yeah. One of the things that does, in fact, distinguish you from those other women who are fine writers in their own right—to your point—one of the things that distinguishes you, Bebe, it seems to me is that you have a unique way of weaving in social themes, social issues with your work. I mean, you can't put a book out in the summer for sisters that doesn't have a little romance in it, and I ain't mad at you for that, but you will weave in some social consciousness with the romance, and you do that very brilliantly. And you've done it in this book and the title, in fact, *72 Hour Hold*, speaks to that, does it not?

Campbell: Well, "72 Hour Hold" is the length of time that a psychiatric facility can hold a mentally ill person against his will if he meets the criteria of a danger to self or danger to others or [is] gravely disabled. And you know you're supposed to write what you know, and I know this world.

I have a mentally ill loved one, a family member, and I've been on a journey with my loved one for about 9 years. So I know about 72 hour holds, I know about conservatorship, I know about the psychotropic drugs, I know about mania. My loved one has bipolar disorder. And I also know about stigma. I know about feeling really, really, really bad and really, really ashamed and not wanting to tell anybody and letting it be my own little deep, dark secret, and I know how useless that is because people with mental illnesses don't keep your secrets.

So I think it's . . . what I wanted to do was to write a good book. I gotta get you from page 1 to page 2 to page 3, and I think I've done that with this. But I'm really—mental illness is my passion now because I've formed a bond with other people who have mentally ill loved ones, many of whom are African American. And we first formed our own support group, then we got involved with the National Alliance for the Mentally Ill and in Southern California, in Los Angeles with some other women we formed a chapter of NAMI, the National Alliance for the Mentally Ill.

And the other thing is I really, really want African Americans to get mental illness out of our collective closet, Tavis, because I keep thinking about *Soul Food*, the movie with Uncle Pete up in the back room, you know, when they slide that dinner tray in and . . . and we have a lot of Uncle Petes in our communities and in communities of color. And we always say, "Well, Uncle Pete is a little strange. Uncle Pete doesn't like to be around people," but we never say Uncle Pete has schizophrenia. And as long as we're in denial about that, we're not gonna get any help for Uncle Pete.

Tavis: I suspect that where writing is concerned—you would know better than I do since you're the *New York Times* bestselling author, not me . . . I suspect that the advice you offered earlier, to write about what you know is good advice.

Campbell: Or what you want to research.

Tavis: Or what you want to research. But I also suspect that it's pretty good advice from your publisher to write what's gonna sell, and to write something that people find interesting and fascinating and you are a novelist, so how does one take a subject like that—that ain't the sexiest thing to write about—

Campbell: No, it's not.

Tavis: And weave it into a novel that's good and that's a page-turner.

Campbell: Well, I was blessed to have an editor who lets me write my passion, and she knew that this was my passion. And, you know, this doesn't—this is a story about a mother, Keri, who has a mentally ill daughter, Trina. Now, Keri's caught up in the middle of a love triangle with her ex-boyfriend and—her ex-husband and her actor boyfriend, and she's got a business and she's got girlfriends and she's got a lot going on in her life, and she's an interesting, complex character. And all of that just sort of stops when she tries to get healing for her child. And she becomes so frustrated with the mental health system that she opts for a radical approach. And that radical approach takes her on a journey that leads to her healing as well as an attempt to get her child healed. So, you know, it's not just about mental illness. I mean, there are pages where you're gonna laugh out loud. And one of the things that when I got into a support group that I allowed myself to do was to laugh at some of the humorous things that occur when you're on a journey with a mentally ill person.

Tavis: I wonder, though, to that point, whether or not it is difficult. On the one hand, I can see it being easier to write about something that you do know. On the other hand, I can see it being difficult even in the context of a novel to actually put that kind of pain on paper, if you will.

Campbell: Well, I don't bring pain to the computer. I think I get through the pain before I approach the computer. In other words, I was walking around with this on my shoulder for years.

Tavis: Is this therapeutic in some way?

Campbell: I think writing is therapeutic for me, yes, because in the frustration of my own dealing with the mental health system, I dreamed up something that I wish existed, but I couldn't find, and this was a radical approach to healing my loved one. So, yeah, getting it on the page and having it really there was therapy for me. And usually writing is not therapy for me. It's work, and it's art. Yeah.

Tavis: Now, I wouldn't be worth my weight as a talk show host if I let that last comment go without going back to pick up on it. So when you suggest that you had to create a world—which is what writers do wonderfully well—to create a world where this mental illness is concerned with regard to your loved one that did not exist, what did you need that you couldn't find that you had to create?

Campbell: Well, I became . . . in searching for healing for my loved one, I became very frustrated with the mental health system. Just the title of the book, *72 Hour Hold*, it takes a good 4 to 6 weeks for the medications that help with schizophrenia or bipolar or depression to get into the person's system. [A] 72 hour hold is like a band-aid for a hemorrhage. You can have someone who meets the criteria—danger to self or danger to others—and when the psychiatric evaluation team arrives at your home, the person pulls it together and presents very well and they go away. So, you know, there's all kinds of frustrations. You've got patients' rights, which I fully understand because there are bad people in the world who would rip off mentally ill people. I understand that, but it's awfully hard to cope with patients' rights when that person is going to be returning to a family member's home. If you're that family member and the 21-year-old says, "Don't tell this person anything," and so you can't get any information and yet you've gotta take that person home at the end of 3 days, that's very difficult as well.

Tavis: Obviously, your books are not just written—not just read—it's certainly written by a black woman—they're not just read by African American women and others, because if they were just read by black women, you wouldn't be on the *New York Times* bestseller list, so obviously, a lot of folk are reading your book even outside of the black community, and yet you mentioned earlier that this is an issue that is of particular importance to you because of the way the black community treats it or maltreats the issue. Does that mean that white folk are like pushing their mentally ill ones out front and saying, "Hey, we deal with this and y'all don't?"

Campbell: No, no. No one, no one wants to say, "I'm not in control of my mind." No one wants to say, "I love someone, I have a family member who is not in control of his mind." Everybody has problems dealing with this. But our problems are greater because we feel the stigma more keenly. We already feel stigmatized by virtue of the color our skins. So then to add something else to this is even more shameful, so we go into denial. The other part of this in terms of why African Americans are less likely to get help—we're less likely to have insurance, we're underinsured, and then we've got—we don't totally trust that medical establishment when that medical establishment is giving out pills for our minds. We still remember Tuskegee [the 1932 study in which the Public Health Service studied four hundred black men with syphilis without telling them what they were being treated for], so we're not totally on board with someone saying there's something wrong with our minds. And yet, I think we've gotta be very, very cautious—I do because there are misdiagnoses and poor diagnosis and no diagnosis, but the danger of not getting help, not getting diagnosed, being in denial is that we wind up in prison, Tavis. So we're disproportionately incarcerated anyway, and there's a disproportionate number of people with mental illnesses in jail. And then what happened a few weeks ago in Los Angeles with the mentally ill man being shot and the baby— the baby being killed, you know, to me that points out that there was a need a long, long time ago, help that this person didn't get.

Tavis: On the back of this book as I close, Maya Angelou, who we all love and respect says, "I am grateful for Bebe Moore Campbell. Campbell fearlessly unveils the pain of loss and the ecstasy of love. Add to that courage, and the graceful ability to write very, very well." So says Dr. Maya Angelou. You've done that in this book. If this book—and I suspect it will do as well as your others have done—so *New York Times* list, get ready for *72 Hour Hold*. If it didn't do as well tackling a subject like this that means a great deal to you, how would that encourage you, discourage you, affect you in your future writings?

Campbell: Well, it affects me as a—you know, as a business person, as an artist business person. You don't get the sales, then, you know, what's the next contract gonna be like— but there's a 2-fold mission on this book tour. I really, really want people to come out of the closet. I really want people to face the issues. I was successful along with NAMI-Inglewood in getting July proclaimed National Minority Mental Health month by Mayor Anthony Williams of Washington, D.C. and Jane Campbell of Cleveland, Ohio. And so, we're gonna have a whole big push. July's going forward to get the churches, get the civic organizations to get some information out there so people are less afraid and less in denial about this. *72 Hour Hold* is my calling card, but it's really just the beginning.

Tavis: Well, there's no denying that Bebe Moore Campbell writes excellent books that we all love to read. *72 Hour Hold* is the most recent one. Bebe, nice to see you.

Campbell: Nice to see you, too, Tavis.

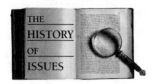

CHAPTER 5

Improving Care
for the Mentally Ill

Chapter Preface

"Fragmented" is the best word to describe the mental health-care system of the United States at the beginning of the twenty-first century. Responsibility for the care and treatment of the mentally ill is split among the federal and state governments, community mental-health centers, and public hospitals. Entitlement programs such as Medicare, Medicaid, Social Security Disability Insurance, and Supplemental Security Income provide medical and economic support for those suffering from mental illness. Many of the mentally ill are also reliant on government programs for the poor, such as public housing programs and food stamps.

This "basket" of diverse programs was created through the efforts of government leaders, mental health-care professionals, reformers, and others who wanted to make it possible for the mentally ill to live in the community. While it does help many individuals achieve that goal, it also has many critics. The critics argue that the disorganized nature of mental health care makes it inefficient and confusing. While in theory it enables the mentally ill to reside in the community, the system is so fragmented that it is difficult for many of the mentally ill to make use of it without help. Despite this important drawback, critics and supporters alike agree that the mentally ill do benefit by living in the community and using the variety of programs available to them.

There are many ways in which the current system can be improved according to psychiatrists, social workers, mental health-care activists, and government leaders. Each argument for improvement reveals a facet of the issue or a problem to overcome. For example, some analysts suggest giving sole responsibility for the care of the mentally ill to the states. This argument is based on the belief that, unlike the federal government, the states know exactly where funds are needed (in urban or rural areas) and how best to allocate them. Others use the issue of homelessness to lobby on behalf of more low-income housing or group homes for the mentally ill. Psychiatrists involved in the treatment of the mentally ill argue in support of court-ordered assisted outpatient treatment for those who do not understand that they are mentally ill and therefore do not accept treatment voluntarily. Doctors and social workers who interact with the mentally ill in the community note how too many of their clients suffer from medical problems such as diabetes or hypertension that go untreated. They suggest adding more medical personnel to existing community mental health clinics.

Veterans returning from duty in Iraq suffering from post-traumatic stress disorder (PTSD) present a new challenge for the nation's mental health-care system. As news reports and individual stories indicate, a soldier's transition from military life to civilian life is often difficult and is made more so because of the psychological trauma of war. Some veterans with PTSD who seek treatment may require short-term care in hospitals or counseling in outpatient clinics. Others may require long periods of hospitalization or psychiatric care. Those who deny a chronic psychological problem risk falling into substance abuse, depression, unemployment, and worse. It is highly likely that at some time or other they will find themselves accessing the mental health-care system either voluntarily or involuntarily.

The following chapter explores this issue and others related to improving care for the mentally ill. How the current imperfect but wide-ranging system evolves to serve mentally ill citizens, their families, and communities is a story that merits following.

A Critique of the Current Mental Health System

Gerald N. Grob

In the 1800s and 1900s, the mentally ill were largely confined to mental institutions far away from the rest of the community. Thus isolated, the patients, their illnesses, and the nature of their care were ignored by the public. "Out of sight, out of mind" best described society's dealings with the mentally ill at this time. With deinstitutionalization and the return of the mentally ill to the community beginning in the mid-1900s, major issues such as housing, outpatient care, and medical care came to the forefront of public discussion. These areas persist in being underfunded by state and federal governments. As a result, the mentally ill— those who most need aid in the tasks of daily living—go underserved by the very mental health-care system that proposes to care for them. This situation is the topic of the following selection by Gerald N. Grob, one of the nation's leading historians of the mental health system. Grob sums up the evolution of the system over the decades and sees the decentralization of the mental health system as one of the main problems in dealing with the chronically mentally ill.

In the early nineteenth century, Americans pursued institutional solutions to resolve complex social problems. To activists such as Horace Mann and Dorothea L. Dix, the mental hospital symbolized the means by which society fulfilled its moral and ethical obligations to mentally ill persons requiring assistance. Such institutions, they insisted, benefited the community, family, and afflicted individual by providing care and treatment irrespective of ability to pay the high costs associated with protracted hospitalization. In the succeeding century the mental hospital became the foundation of a policy that guaranteed access to care and treatment for the mentally ill. From modest beginnings, the number and size of mental hospitals increased with each passing decade. At their peak they contained a resident population in excess of half a million and accounted for a substantial proportion of state welfare budgets.

Paradoxically, a century later public mental hospitals had come to be perceived as the problem rather than the solution. At the end of World War II many institutions were suffering from nearly two decades of neglect. A deteriorated physical plant, shortages of psychiatrists and other staff, overcrowding, and a preoccupation with the need to provide custodial care for large numbers of chronically mentally ill persons were characteristic. Faced with an institutional policy that appeared inhumane and bankrupt, a coalition of professional and lay activists launched a crusade to transform mental health policy. Their goal was simple but radical, namely, to begin a process that would culminate in the replacement of traditional mental hospitals with new forms of community care and treatment.

Mental Health Services Expand

The dramatic policy shifts of the postwar decades had important consequences. [Director of the National Institute of Mental Health] Robert H. Felix's crusade to confer legitimacy upon mental health services and to incorporate them within the framework of health care was largely successful. Community psychiatric and psychological services grew rapidly; general hospitals expanded their psychiatric capabilities; and acute services for the severely mentally ill expanded both quantitatively and qualitatively. Public mental hospitals were relieved of the burden of caring for large numbers of chronic and especially aged patients, which facilitated their conversion into more active treatment centers. Finally, mental health services grew somewhat less stigmatized, thus enhancing their popularity and use among both nonmentally and mentally ill groups.

The consequences of human activities, however, tend to be complex and unpredictable; ambiguity—not clarity or consistency—is often characteristic. This is especially true for the changes in the mental health system since World War II. Prior to 1940 the focus of public policy had been almost exclusively on the severely and chronically mentally ill. This policy was based on the assumption that society had an obligation to provide such unfortunate persons with both care and treatment in public mental hospitals. The policies adopted during and after the 1960s rested on quite different assumptions. That public mental hospitals continued to play an important role is indisputable. The creation of a decentralized and heterogeneous system of services, however, diminished their relative significance. Equally important, the target population became more diffuse and variegated: the mental health system was no longer concerned solely with the severely and chronically mentally ill. Even those professionals involved in providing services were less likely to deal with a group that presented formidable and sometimes insoluble problems. Ironically, the growing availability, variety, and popularity of mental health services sometimes worked to the detriment of those most in need of assistance.

Care for a Defined vs. a Broad Population

Perhaps one of the most striking results of the postwar shift in policy was the severing of the traditional and previously unbreakable ties between care and treatment. Despite monumental shortcomings, mental hospitals had provided at least a basic level of care for many individuals incapable of functioning as independent and self-reliant human beings. Moreover, mental hospital care had derived legitimacy from its identification with medical science. Thus these institutions did not have to bear the burden of being tied to a welfare system grounded in part on the belief that dependency was self-inflicted, and that poverty, misfortune, and illnesses were consequences of character deficiencies rather than environmental or biological circumstances.

The community mental health policies that emerged during the postwar decades inadvertently distorted priorities by strengthening the distinction between care and treatment. Admittedly, these policies paid rhetorical homage to the need for care. Reality, however, was quite different. The main focus was on providing therapeutic services in outpatient settings to a broad, rather than a defined, population. Consequently, the social and human needs of the most severely and especially chronically mentally ill—particularly assistance in dealing with the subsistence tasks of daily life—were often ignored or overlooked. The identification of mental health policy with therapeutic services was understandable, given the obvious advantages of being included within the medical health care system. Caring and support services, by way of contrast, were affiliated with a welfare system that by the 1970s and 1980s was under attack by a political constituency bent on diminishing governmental responsibilities and activities.

The subtle shifts in the mental health system were to have tragic consequences for many chronically and severely mentally ill persons most in need of assistance. In the 1970s and 1980s they were often cast adrift in communities without access to support services or the basic necessities of life. For such persons the transition from an institutional to a community-based system proved devastating. By the 1980s the presence of homeless mentally ill persons in many communities served as a stark reminder that the new mental health policies had negative as well as positive consequences.

Not Facing Up to Complexities of Life

In their desire to improve the lives of the severely mentally ill, psychiatric and lay activists had helped to lay the foundation for a new policy. Like others before them, they dismissed out of hand the experiences of the past. A peculiar blend of indignation at the continued existence of mental hospitals and a faith in a professionally grounded ideology combined to lay the groundwork for ending what to them was an obsolete and bankrupt policy. Ironically, overstated claims, enthusiasm for change, and an inability to appreciate the complexity of non-institutional life for many severely and chronically mentally ill persons led these activists to overlook the difficulties that impeded the creation of support systems capable of providing care outside of institutions.

Human triumphs invariably incorporate elements of tragedy as well. The generation that reached maturity during and after the 1940s firmly believed that the adoption of new mental health policies would lead to dramatic improvements. Their efforts played a major role in reshaping the mental health system by shifting the focus away from an institutional system plagued with severe problems. At the same time they sometimes failed to understand the human and social needs of the very persons they wanted to help, and they consistently overestimated their ability to shape administrative mechanisms, institutions, and policies. Although a broad constituency benefited from their innovative policies, many who required the most assistance—especially the chronically mentally ill—lost. More than a century and a half after a system of public mental hospitals was created, Americans had yet to define a mental health policy that integrated decent and humane *care* with access to medical services for severely and chronically mentally ill persons.

A Blueprint for Change

E. Fuller Torrey

Providing care for the chronically mentally ill will continue to demand large infusions of money from federal, state, and local governments according to E. Fuller Torrey, the author of the following excerpt from his book Out of the Shadows. *Torrey is a research psychiatrist at the Neuroscience Center of the National Institute of Mental Health and is a critic of the nation's mental health system.*

In the excerpt Torrey explains why he is opposed to the way the system operates and recommends specific economic, legal, and ideological changes that he believes will help the chronically mentally ill. One of his proposals is to give the states the sole authority for planning and paying for mental health-care services. A point of controversy that places Torrey in opposition to civil rights advocates is his belief that involuntary treatment for a portion of the mentally ill population is necessary.

Until research provides more definitive answers regarding causes and treatments, we will continue to be faced with providing psychiatric services for an estimated 5.6 million people who are mentally ill. . . . We know how to provide services that are high quality, humane, and cost-effective, but for a variety of reasons we do not do so. The following summary highlights my major recommendations . . . for achieving such services.

- *The economic solution: Single responsibility funding.* Cost-shifting between federal and state, and state and local governments is the single largest cause of the mental illness crisis.

- Single responsibility funding is the proposed solution. The states would be given authority for planning and for financing services, although the funds may be derived from federal and local as well as state taxes. The states would also be held accountable for treatment outcomes, and this would continue to be true even if the states subcontract for the services with county or city governments or with private sector providers.

- Block grants of federal funds to the states are consistent with single responsibility funding as long as the states are required to spend those funds on the target population and treatment outcomes are being measured.

- The measurement of treatment outcomes is mandatory for solving the present crisis. If treatment outcomes are being measured then performance contracting becomes possible.

- We do not yet know the optimal system of financial incentives for ensuring quality services for people who are mentally ill. Therefore, it is appropriate to encourage state and local governments to try different arrangements, using public, private nonprofit and for-profit resources, as long as treatment outcomes are being measured and the outcomes of the various financial arrangements are being assessed. At the same time, the dismal record to date of the for-profit sector in providing services for individuals with severe mental illnesses should be acknowledged and makes it more likely that definitive solutions will come from the non-profit sector.

Involuntary Treatment

- *The legal solution: Recognition of the need for involuntary treatment.* Since approximately half of all persons with severe mental illnesses have impaired insight because of their illnesses and therefore do not recognize their need for treatment, a substantial number of the mentally ill will have to be treated involuntarily if they are going to be treated at all. The failure to do so is a major contributor to this crisis.

- Involuntary commitment laws for hospitalization and treatment should be based not only on dangerousness to self or others, but also on the need for treatment. As measures of insight improve and scales with good inter-rated reliability are developed, a measure of insight should also be included in commitment criteria.

- In assessing a mentally ill person's need for involuntary treatment, the person's past history should always be considered. Special attention should be directed to the person's history of violent behavior, alcohol and drug abuse, and noncompliance with medication since these are known to be the major predictors of future violent behavior.

- Conditional release, guardianships, and outpatient commitment should be available and used for mentally ill persons who are in need of involuntary treatment and who can live successfully in the community as long as they take their medication.

- Interstate reciprocity should be established and enforced for mentally ill persons who are involuntarily committed to treatment in one state.

- The federally funded Protection and Advocacy program should be abolished.

- For mentally ill persons who also abuse alcohol or drugs, SSI, SSDI, and VA [Supplemental Security Income, Social Security Disability Insurance, and Veterans Administration] benefits should be paid directly to a representative payee who is directly connected to the person's treatment program. The person's benefits should become part of the treatment plan to reduce the person's alcohol or drug abuse. The benefits would therefore change from being part of the problem to being part of the solution.

- SSI, SSDI, and VA benefits for mentally ill persons should be standardized. Consideration should also be given to establishing two levels of disability—partial and total—to encourage people to work who are capable of doing so.

- A small percentage of the mentally ill are not capable of living in the community because of the severity of their symptoms, their propensity toward violent behavior, their concurrent alcohol or drug abuse, or their nonresponsiveness to all available medication. It should be acknowledged that long-term hospitalization is both appropriate and necessary for these patients.

- *The ideological solution: Divorce mental illness from mental health.* The continuum concept, which has dominated twentieth-century thinking about mental disorders, is an important cause of the mental illness crisis. Severe mental illnesses are *not* merely one end of a mental health continuum. It is therefore necessary to return to the nineteenth-century idea that these illnesses are in a different category from problems of mental health. A divorce of mental illness from mental health could be accomplished by the following.

- A National Brain Research Institute should be formed by a merger of the National Institute of Mental Health and the National Institute of Neurological Disorders and Stroke.

- State departments of mental health should be abolished. People with severe mental illnesses should be the responsibility of the state department of health and should receive services in the same clinics as do patients with other neurological disorders.

- In medical schools, the departments of psychiatry and neurology should merge. The joint department would train neuropsychiatrists who would be specialists in neurological disorders, mental illnesses, and other nonsurgical disorders of the brain.

- Since medical resources are finite, a system of prioritization should be established in which severe mental illnesses are prioritized along with other medical disorders. A combination of criteria could be used including structural and functional brain abnormalities, functional impairment, likelihood of benefit from treatment, economic cost-benefit, social cost-benefit and fairness.

- Since severe mental illnesses would no longer be part of a mental health spectrum they should no longer be politicized.

Gaining Insight into Lack of Insight

Jim Reiser

Many mentally ill persons refuse treatment because they believe there is nothing wrong with them. Psychologists call this anosognosia or "lack of awareness" and pinpoint it as one of the main challenges in dealing with a person who is mentally ill. Doctors, social workers, law enforcement officers, and caretakers who deal with the mentally ill on a daily basis must find ways to communicate with the unaware in order to get them to accept help. Finding avenues of communication with the mentally ill is the topic of the article that follows. The author, Jim Reiser, writing for the Web site of the New York City affiliate of the National Alliance on Mental Illness, argues that recent programs and approaches fail on all grounds because they either overlook the issue of lack of awareness or see the mentally ill as primarily patients. Reiser then presents his own methodology for dealing with lack of awareness. His approach is based on his experiences with a sibling's illness.

Anosognosia ("anasugNOHZeeah") or lack of awareness of one's mental illness is another biologically based symptom like hallucinations or delusions. Once we acknowledge this, a realistic strategy for coping becomes apparent. Implications for family members are favorable.

Sadly, the mental health service system has not demonstrated an understanding of this symptom in most of its programs. Individuals suffering from anosognosia are frequently homeless, incarcerated, noncompliant, violent, refuse treatment, and they are often caught in the revolving door of a fragmented mental health system and become candidates for

Jim Reiser, "Service System Lacks Insight into Lack of Insight," *NAMI-NYCMETRO/ naminycmetro.org*. Reproduced by permission.

Kendra's Law [a New York law that created a framework for court-ordered assisted outpatient treatment].

How are programs meeting the needs of those who have no awareness they are ill? Apparently they are not. In fact, Kendra's Law can be seen as the frustrated public reaction to the failure of the system to meet these needs. We end up in court because the mental health service system has proven unable to help these people.

An Assumption and an Approach

Ill person not engaged—Newer "progressive" programs frequently fail to meaningfully help individuals suffering from anosognosia. For example, peer programs, which represent a wonderful development in the field, do not meet the needs of the "unaware" because these programs do not engage them. The programs assume in their design that the peer candidate has an understanding of their illness. Otherwise the person would not meet the criteria of peer. The philosophy of this service orientation is based on engaging the "motivated consumer." The success of this program is linked to the voluntary and active involvement of the consumer.

But what about those "consumers" who are not motivated because they are unaware they are consumers? The 40–50% of the chronically mentally ill suffering from anosognosia are by definition not part of the peer movement and therefore not served by peer-directed programming. While these more progressive programs fail the unaware, the other end of the spectrum is also flawed. The Treatment Advocacy Center's [TAC, an organization that advocates for the elimination of barriers to effective treatment for severe mental illness] approach promotes the medical model to such a degree that it gets in the way of engaging the unaware individual. During TAC director Dr. E. Fuller Torrey's Q&A at NAMI's [National Alliance on Mental Illness] September general meeting he said, "there are only patients and not clients." This frame of reference eliminates the common ground for engaging the unaware into a productive relationship.

Collaborate, don't lecture—I know from a long history of coping with my brother's illness that if I were still thinking of him only in this medical frame, he would not be doing as well as he is right now. Only after I acknowledged that I needed to collaborate with him rather than lecture him about treatment did I "get" him to receive treatment. It was only after I started practicing the "LEAP" strategy outlined in Dr. Xavier Amador's book *I'm Not Sick, I Don't Need Help: Helping the Severely Mentally Ill Accept Treatment,* that we moved ahead. If we still conceive of our loved ones only as patients, I contend we can't even start to "Listen & Empathize," or be anywhere near on our way to "Agreeing" on anything.

One Program That Listens

While most community programs fail those with anosognosia, there are signs of hope. One of these is Pathways to Housing, an eight-year-old program in the city that intentionally separates housing from treatment. Sam Tsemberis Ph.D., Executive Director, explained that separating the clinical from housing was the key to not only engaging the homeless mentally ill but also keeping them in the program. Most other community housing programs require candidates to be "housing ready," i.e. already compliant regarding chemical dependencies on the one hand and medical treatment on the other. Pathways does not require this.

The program is succeeding with those who are unaware because it offers something up front that is perhaps the most meaningful to them: personal housing. The only requirements are that the individual must visit with a coordinator at least twice a month, and work with the coordinator in managing the individual's money. There are no other requirements, no MICA [mentally ill chemical abusers] or medical treatment requirements, nothing.

Listening and empathizing—This program has, in effect, adopted the LEAP strategy because it starts by listening and empathizing with the client. Pathways partners with the client after getting the client to agree with some fairly easy and straightforward requirements. Eventually most clients engage the coordinators so that the number of visits increases. This active relationship works to encourage and engage the client and encourages treatment. As we all know in working with mental illness, this program still faces the realities of psychotic breaks and "noncompliant" behavior, but Pathways holds the apartment for the individual while he is in hospital treatment. The one statistic that jumps out here is that Pathways to Housing has a retention rate of 85%! This is incredible given the treatment-resistant homeless population it serves.

Treating the Medical Problems of the Mentally Ill

Ralph Aquila, M.D., Thomas Malamud, Thomas Sweet, and John D. Kelleher

Homelessness, lack of awareness, noncompliance with treatment plans, drug addiction, and alcoholism are some of the most pressing problems of the mentally ill. Access to medical care is another. According to the authors of the following article, too many severely mentally ill persons suffer from poor nutrition, mistrust doctors and hospitals, and wait until symptoms of disease are advanced before seeking help. All of these factors contribute to the dire medical state of the mentally ill.

The authors (a professor of psychiatry, a director of special projects at the Center for Reintegration, the director of special projects at Fountain House, and a Fountain House member, respectively) describe the health behaviors that put the mentally ill at risk and explain how their storefront facility in New York City provides access to mental health services and medical treatment. The storefront is part of Fountain House, a community-based support system established in 1948 for the recovery of mentally ill persons and their return to the community.

As recent events, news stories, and evaluations performed at Fountain House have illustrated, men and women with serious and persistent mental illness (generally schizophrenia, bipolar, or other affective disorders), particularly those who are or have been homeless—roughly 60% of the Fountain House membership—are substantially more likely to have comorbid [other additional] medical illnesses than the general population.

Fountain House, for those unaware of this model of psychiatric rehabilitation, is a community-based, comprehensive support system established in 1948 by patients and volunteers from Rockland (New York) State Hospital. The first program of its kind in the United States, the Fountain House's innovative and consumer-centered model for recovery has been replicated throughout the United States and abroad. Since 1948, Fountain House has pioneered and developed extensive programs for facilitating the social and vocational adjustment of men and women following hospitalization in public and private mental hospitals and has served over 16,000 individuals through a comprehensive array of accessible, integrated, and long-term systems of care. There are now Fountain House Model Programs in close to 40 countries around the world, and approximately 200 in the United States alone.

With the advent of "atypical" antipsychotic medications (such as clozapine, risperidone, olanzapine, quetiapine, and others) the overt symptomatology of patients is likely to lessen, many times becoming transparent to the eye (eg, no herky-jerky motions, involuntary movements, extreme sedation). This result does not mean that the effects of the newer medications avoid the presence of comorbidities (eg, obesity).

Why Substandard Care?

An innovative approach to meeting this challenge is currently being tested in a joint effort between 2 New York City facilities—Fountain House and the Saint Luke's/Roosevelt Hospital Center (STL/R). What we are addressing in this article is the well-documented fact that these men and women are more likely to receive substandard or no medical care, especially in urban areas. There are several reasons for this deplorable situation:

- The lifestyle of people with serious and persistent mental illness often includes poor nutrition (most live on an income significantly below the federal poverty line, leaving little money for food), exposure to infectious diseases (including TB [tuberculosis], STDs [sexually transmitted diseases], and HIV), and high rates of substance abuse, current or historical (over 65% at Fountain House).

- People with mental illness typically do not seek out primary medical prevention, and often ignore early symptoms of medical illness when they occur. They generally have a mistrust of doctors and medical institutions, and, therefore, they often do not seek medical treatment until they are in the advanced stages of an illness. Further, medical professionals often view people with mental illness as unreliable reporters, and often discount the symptoms they describe. . . .

Bridging the Treatment Gap

The treatment gap for people with mental illness is one of the most important issues in mental health today. The magnitude and burden of mental and behavioral disorders are common, affecting 20% to 25% of all people at some time during their life. They are also universal—affecting all countries and societies, and individuals at all ages. Mental disorders have a large direct and indirect economic impact on societies, particularly service costs. Perhaps more important, the negative impact on the quality of life of individuals and families is massive. It is estimated that, in 1990, mental and neurologic disorders accounted for over 15% of the total "disability-adjusted life years" (DALYs) lost due to all diseases and injuries. That study also estimated that by the year 2020, the burden of these disorders will have increased significantly. Yet only a small minority of all those presently affected receive any treatment.

In 1992, as part of a new housing initiative by Fountain House, a supervised residence for homeless, mentally ill single adults was opened, with psychiatric services provided by STL/R. This relationship grew over the next 3 years, leading to the leasing of a storefront near Fountain House where individuals could easily access mental health services. It became clear that with the population being served (primarily homeless or recently homeless), many individuals were in desperate need of primary medical care, which was largely not easily accessible. This led to the expansion of the storefront to include a PCP [primary care physician]. Having operated the storefront for 11 years, we believe it now qualifies as an evidence-based practice that must be shared with the medical and non-medical community; following is a brief description of who we are, the approach being utilized, some examples, and where we would like to go in the future.

As the first program of its kind in the United States, Fountain House endeavors to remain on the cutting edge of innovative and consumer-centered models for recovery, such as addressing the physical wellness of patients that are generally seen as being affected exclusively psychiatrically. Fountain House is an "intentional community" based on the belief that those men and women (hereafter referred to as "members," not patients, clients, consumers, or any other label) suffering from serious and persistent mental illness can and will achieve normal life goals when provided opportunities, time, support, and audience (fellowship). A complete description of all Fountain House programs and services can be found at www.fountainhouse.org and elsewhere.

Special mention must be made of how the Fountain House community views medication, psychiatric, dual diagnoses, and medical needs, none of which are offered as part of its continuum of services. Fountain House plays an important role in helping participants maintain themselves on prescribed medication and in assuring that they continue to have access to the clinical treatment care they need.

For many, there is the opportunity to receive a number of these services at a nearby storefront facility operated by STL/R. Currently, the staff includes 3 part-time psychiatrists, 1 part-time PCP, 1 part-time nurse, and clerical staffing. In addition, a variety of other services are available in the storefront, including the following groups: (1) Weight Watchers; (2) double-trouble meetings (a combination of traditional Alcoholics Anonymous 12-step meetings and the understanding for a need for psychotropic medication, started in 1994 by a group of consumers in New York state; prior to this, Alcoholics Anonymous models frowned on psychotropic medications); (3) smoking cessation meetings; (4) diabetes education and support groups; and (5) nutritional education. Storefront hours are 9 AM to 5 PM, Monday through Friday, and several evenings for the various self-help groups. Because of the presence of the storefront facility, access to various services both in- and outpatient at St Luke's/Roosevelt Hospital is easily facilitated.

The Care Provided

To begin addressing the problems identified above, which affect some 100,000 men and women in New York City, the Fountain House-STL/R storefront partnership attempts to deliver community-based primary medical care to some 500 members with serious and persistent mental illness. The following are some of the major characteristics of the care provided by the storefront:

- Services which are close to home, including general hospital care for acute admissions, and long-term residential facilities in the community;

- Interventions related to disabilities as well as symptoms;

- Treatment and care specific to the diagnosis and needs of each individual;

- A wide range of services which address the needs of people with mental and behavioral disorders;

- Services which are coordinated between mental health professionals and community agencies;

- Ambulatory rather than static services, including those which can offer home treatment;

- Partnership with caregivers that remains consistent over time, helping to meet individual needs.

The treatment gap for most mental disorders is high, but in the poor population it is indeed massive. People with serious and persistent mental illness have traditionally been perceived as too disabled to participate in mainstream society. Advances in diagnosis, treatment, and more effective psychotropic medications, as well as access to community-based rehabilitation programs, have begun to change this picture. Long-term outcome studies and first person accounts demonstrate that people with the most serious of mental illnesses can dramatically alter their lives through what has been called a recovery process.

Key to the success of this process, we believe, is the innovative device identified as the Rehabilitation Alliance. This approach to community-based programming for members who have experienced serious and persistent mental illness consists, at a minimum, of a [Fountain House] member, physician, and at least one other—either a clubhouse staff person or another member. In this alliance, each individual plays a different, but coequal role. The goal of the alliance is the provision of vocational, social, educational, residential, mental, and physical health services along with the time and support needed to fulfill these opportunities. . . .

The following 2 examples illustrate what this alliance can accomplish:

Jack is a 65-year-old member who was given access to the storefront PCP on the recommendation of his rehabilitation alliance. As a result, a cancerous growth on his kidney was detected early enough that surgical intervention has led to remission for the past 2 years.

Brigitte, a 40-year-old member, who had not seen a PCP for over 10 years, was, on the recommendation of the rehabilitation alliance, referred to the storefront PCP. Routine examination led to the discovery of a diseased gall bladder, which was removed some 18 months ago, aiding Brigitte to resume normal activities almost immediately.

Both Jack and Brigitte admit to aversion to seeking out medical care because of prior negative experiences.

This unique approach to improving the psychiatric and medical well-being of men and women with serious mental illness is a revolutionary one, just as the original Fountain House was in its inception. It represents both a challenge and a potential solution to the problems articulated in this paper; unfortunately a challenge that has yet to be accepted in either the medical or psychiatric field by most practitioners, despite the success attained over the past 11 years through the storefront partnership with Fountain House.

Negotiating the Maze
of Social Programs

Richard G. Frank and Sherry A. Glied

The United States has made great strides in improving the quality of mental health care in the past forty years. The appearance of a new generation of drugs for example, gives the mentally ill improved chances of clinical recovery. The rights of the mentally ill are protected under law, and advocacy organizations exist to help them have a voice in government. The mainstreaming of the mentally ill into the community has given rise to a web of local, state, and federal social service programs that ideally provide lifelong mental health-care treatment and economic support. In order to accomplish this lifelong support for the mentally ill, states have to fit mentally ill people into service categories recognized by mainstream insurance and social programs. The ill and/or their families are required to negotiate the programs in order to get treatment and to access programs. According to mental health system analysts Richard G. Frank and Sherry A. Glied, negotiating this web of programs is extremely difficult or impossible for the severely mentally ill. While applauding mainstreaming as a whole, Frank and Glied see the need for a new federal agency to oversee the various programs now administered by the states and federal government.

The overarching deficiency of mainstreaming [treating the mentally ill in society, as opposed to within an institution] is that it abandons the public responsibility for mental health care and the well-being of people with severe mental illnesses to a fragmented array of public programs that are run out of a large number of distinct federal, state, and local government bureaucracies. This fragmentation is in itself unexceptional. Under the best of circumstances, social insurance programs in the United States present potential beneficiaries with a complex array of inconsistent rules. For people with severe mental disorders, whose illnesses inherently put them at a particular disadvantage in negotiating the maze of social program requirements, the fragmented social insurance system has especially deleterious effects on well-being.

How the presence of mental illnesses of different types affects eligibility, program requirements (e.g., work effort), and duration of benefits is highly variable. Those programs with an exceptionally high representation of people with mental illness, such as Medicaid, sometimes recognize special circumstances associated with mental illnesses. Most do not.

The policy challenge is to encourage the integration of people with mental disorders into the mainstream of U.S. society and social programs, at the same time recognizing unique features of their circumstances that federal, state, local, and private social and medical insurance programs must take into account to effectively serve them. This goal requires a new model of stewardship for the mental health system.

A New Model of Stewardship

Historically, public mental hospitals and SMHAs [state mental health agencies] formed the core of the mental health care delivery and support system. These identifiable agencies and institutions were visible to mental health care consumers, their families, and their advocates. SMHAs could be and were held politically accountable for mental health care. They were conduits for the voices of people with mental disorders and those interested in their well-being. They were the foundation of a mental health care system based on exceptionalism. Yet the cost of that specialized focal point was a system that had little general political support and was chronically underfunded.

As these institutions have lost financial authority over the past three decades, the challenge of creating a new model of stewardship has been an enduring topic for policy proposals. Most proposals during the 1980s and 1990s recommended expanding the reach of public mental health agencies at either the state or the local level. The idea was to assign to a single public agency responsibility for managing diverse funding streams, treatment, and other forms of support and care for severely mentally ill people who are aided by public health, social, and income support programs. Looking backward, however, we can see that the track record of initiatives that placed a public mental health agency in a centralized planning role has been poor. These initiatives invariably became less able to maintain funding growth because they required continuous special pleadings; they became rigid because the voices of specialty mental health providers and mental health advocates were the only ones heard in decisions about program design; and they became progressively narrower because the specialty mental health sector frequently is limited in its expertise about the delivery of other human services (e.g., housing).

We should not reject mainstreaming, even for seriously mentally ill populations. The institutional foundations for future progress for people with serious mental disorders are the same as those that proved successful in the past—large, broad-based social and health insurance programs as well as the mainstream bio-medical research enterprise. Medicaid, Medicare, and Social Security are generally popular. They address a wide set of expanding needs in U.S. society. Even Medicaid, long associated with politically vulnerable means-tested social programs, has managed to grow in significance and continues to enjoy considerable political support. The National Institutes of Health and the pharmaceutical industry have produced a series of major advances in treatment of mental disorders. We need to build a new stewardship structure that is consistent with mainstreaming.

A Presence in the Federal Government Is Needed

This institutional structure needs to have several distinctive characteristics. First, the financial center of gravity in care and support of people with mental illness has moved to the federal level. Medicare, the Food Stamp program, SSDI [Social Security Disability Insurance] and much housing policy are purely federal. Most large employer health benefit plans are regulated exclusively by the federal government. Medicaid, SSI [Supplemental Security Income] and welfare are partnerships between the federal government and the states, with the federal government often establishing overarching rules that govern the allocation of funds. State governments remain critically important in mental health service delivery, and, as President Bush's New Freedom Commission (2003) suggested, mental health needs within states require enhanced governance. In addition, however, effective stewardship will require an institutional presence in the federal government. It is in the federal bureaucracy that a stewardship function will have the greatest opportunity for policy influence.

Second, progress has come through mainstream programs. Thus, a new federal stewardship institution should not administer or finance specialized mental health programs. Rather, it should take the form of introducing the concerns of people with serious and persistent mental illness and some corresponding elements of exceptionalism into larger social and health insurance agencies. It should advocate for the interests of people with mental illness and coordinate services among programs and across systems.

Third, many of the gains of the past fifty years have come about through the concerted efforts of people with mental illness and their families and supporters. A new agency should provide a locus for lobbying and advocacy efforts. It should channel the ideas and concerns of people with mental illness to the appropriate programmatic bureaucracy.

Fourth, the new institution needs to have a position within the federal bureaucracy that will provide it with authority. This implies that it should report directly to the president, rather than be subsumed within one of the departments or agencies whose activities it should be critiquing and coordinating. It further implies that the agency have some budgetary control. Though it would be inappropriate for an institution without programmatic authority to develop its own budgets, the new institution should have the ability to question or even veto agency appropriations focused on mental health.

The federal government contains a variety of structures that serve similar purposes, coordinating policy across diverse federal agencies. Over the past fifty years, such coordinating agencies have proliferated. The National Security Agency, the Council of Economic Advisors, and the National Economic Council all represent organizations aimed at assisting in coordination of information and decision making. All are advisory to the president and obtain their influence from that role, but they do not have any budgetary authority and do not influence policy at the state or local level.

A Model for a New Agency

One existing government entity that might serve as a model for housing a new mental health stewardship function is the Office of National Drug Control Policy (ONDCP). The ONDCP is charged with coordinating the array of federal agencies that participate in drug control to ensure that the activities of those agencies are consistent with the national drug control strategy. The ONDCP was created by 1988 legislation outlining a national drug control policy. The ONDCP was given a number of duties and several specific powers. Its first duty was to develop a national drug control strategy. Its second was to develop a budget for implementing that strategy. Its third duty was to oversee and coordinate implementation of the strategy by federal agencies. . . .

A federal agency to oversee the range of programs and regulations that may affect people with mental illness would be a significant step forward. It would institutionalize a voice for mental illness within the federal bureaucracy and enable mainstream policies to be tailored to the needs of people with mental illness. But a federal agency alone will not lift people with mental illness from poverty or ensure that their basic human needs are met.

Adding another layer of bureaucracy rarely improves the functioning of government. In this case, however, the proposed bureaucracy creates a locus of interest and responsibility at the federal level, where none now exists. Though the new agency may have limited capacity to take action, it should help in reorienting advocacy and interest group activity away from the states, whose powers are receding in this arena, and toward the federal government. Moreover, it should for the first time insert into the existing federal bureaucracy a voice for mental health.

People with serious and persistent mental illness can and do benefit from mainstream programs. Yet it is entirely feasible for society to do better still by this severely disadvantaged population.

Community-Based Care for the Mentally Ill Needs to Be Strongly Regulated

Patrik Jonsson

The deinstitutionalization of the mentally ill over the past thirty years and their placement in community-based housing marked a revolution in how states care for their most needy citizens, according to Patrik Jonsson, a staff writer for the Christian Science Monitor. *In the following selection, Jonsson reports on the risks involved in placing the mentally ill in group homes that may be poorly equipped and understaffed. The lack of safety devices such as sprinkler systems placed the residents of one residential home in Missouri at great risk when a fire broke out. Ten people lost their lives as a result of the blaze.*

As Jonsson points out, states face a dilemma about how strictly they should enforce regulations. States may turn a blind eye to deficiencies in group homes because these private operators generally do a good job of caretaking for small federal and state payouts. Also, in many states, group homes represent the only housing alternatives available to the mentally ill. In Missouri alone, 22 percent of the mentally disabled population has been moved into eleven hundred community homes since 2000.

The deadly fire at a group home for the elderly and mentally disabled in an Ozarks town Monday [November 27, 2006,] may hold lessons for a country that is closing many of its state institutions in favor of private community-based facilities.

Nine clients as well as one staff member perished Monday at the Anderson Guest House in Anderson, Mo., which housed

32 residents and two overnight staff. Early worries of arson faded Tuesday. But for Missourians horrified by the blaze, questions linger.

A main concern is why the state didn't require the group home to be equipped with a sprinkler system, especially since people there have difficulty moving around.

That, mental health professionals say, points to problems in both state funding and regulatory oversight, which vary from state to state. But a common problem across the country is that group homes are taking in more difficult clients with needs and requirements that many smaller facilities are not equipped to handle.

Dealing with People with Significant Disabilities

"The level of disability is more significant in these congregate community settings than people had anticipated, and we have to examine that across the country in how prepared we are for these people to come to group homes," says Dave Richard, executive director of The ARC of North Carolina, an advocacy group for people with mental disabilities in Raleigh.

For three decades, the US has been in the midst of a seismic movement in how states care for the mentally ill. Helped along by movies such as *One Flew Over the Cuckoo's Nest*, that depicted abuses possible in isolated state wards, the 411,215 mentally disabled Americans and tens of thousands more classified as mentally ill have trickled out of institutions and into community-based facilities, many of them group homes in residential areas.

Nationally, the number of mentally disabled people in large institutions has dropped from 22 percent to 16 percent [from 2001 to 2006].

Echoes of a 1999 US Supreme Court decision resounds through the debate. Justices ruled in *Olmstead v. L.C.* that states must move patients into the least restrictive housing possible for their condition, which has significantly hastened the flow of patients from large institutions into smaller ones, and, ultimately, into their own apartments.

Ethically, it's the right thing, experts agree. But some states had concerns that deinstitutionalization would lead to problems. That has borne true in some respects, including problems with quality of care, safety and availability of services, and trained staff in some smaller care homes.

Not Enough Support to Help Clients

"States may be reluctant to get on board with [deinstitutionalization] because there are concerns that there aren't enough supports to help [clients] be in the community," says Jessica Jonikas, a director at the Center on Mental Health Services and Research Policy in Chicago.

Another factor, says Mr. Richard, is that many higher-functioning patients, per *Olmstead*, have been moved into independent-living situations, leaving the most difficult patients now transferring out of state hospitals. Depending on how their conditions are classified, many rely solely on state aid except for a small Social Security supplement. Societal costs plunge from $130,000 for institutional settings to $60,000 for community settings, according to amicus briefs filed in the *Olmstead* case.

"We believe that people should live in the community, but the ethical question is how you balance the risk of events like what happened in Missouri against the risks of places where people live in [state institutional] settings," says Richard. "It's really the funding that isn't designed to support people with more significant disabilities."

That means that regulators tend not to be tough on private operators doing, for the most part, admirable and necessary work. For example, the Anderson Guest House was permitted to operate without putting in a sprinkler system since it was built before 1980, the year a system was required by state law. It was determined to be too expensive to retrofit the building.

"There's always tension between holding to the letter of the regulations versus allowing these places to operate, because there isn't much else out there" in the way of options for troubled clients, says Judith Gran, an attorney with the Public Interest Law Center in Philadelphia.

To be sure, 22 percent of the mentally disabled population in Missouri have been shifted from institutions into 1,100 community facilities around the state since 2000, according to the Research and Training Center on Community Living in Minneapolis.

It's not clear yet how, or if, difficulties adjusting to that shift played into the tragic events that unfolded as a quick moving fire shot 30-foot flames from doors and windows in Anderson. The state is promising a serious and thorough review of its funding and licensing procedures.

"It's safe to say that legislators, when they return to Jefferson City, will be looking at regulations regarding this horrific incident," says Brian Hauswirth, a spokesman for Missouri Gov. Matt Blunt.

Providing Mental Health Care for Soldiers in Iraq

Trish Wood

The mental health-care community in the United States is going to have to deal with the psychological ailments of returning Iraq War veterans for years to come. Like returning veterans of previous wars, many of the soldiers who fought in Iraq suffer from post-traumatic stress disorder (PTSD), an anxiety disorder that can occur following the experiencing or witnessing of a traumatic event such as might take place during war. While most survivors of such trauma return to normal with the passage of time, others do not. Some victims of PTSD have stress reactions that worsen as days, weeks, and months pass. Individuals with PTSD may develop serious disorders such as depression or substance abuse and require therapy and/or hospitalization.

The following excerpt is taken from an oral history of the Iraq War. In it a psychology specialist stationed in Iraq recounts her experiences working with and counseling soldiers who live with the daily stressors of the war zone. She finds them particularly vulnerable because of their youth, their separation from family, and their often troubled backgrounds.

I knew from my experience in the army before I became a psych specialist in the National Guard that a lot of young people who come into the military have issues. Being in that environment, and not having any real friends when they come in and no family close by, they just get into a lot of trouble. I had lived in the barracks because I was single, and I noticed there was a lot of drinking, a lot of people just sleeping around, and at that young age it seemed that they were looking for comfort and connection. When you go into the army you are taken away from all your support. I knew I wanted to help these people.

Looking at myself, I came from a small town and a divorced family. My father was an alcoholic, and I think other people like me joined the military to escape and start a new life. However, when you get in, so many people are like that that you can connect with the wrong group instead of taking advantage of what the military has to offer. They can easily be sucked into the alcoholism and the solitude of the military. . . .

The way I ended up in Iraq was that I had just come back on active duty after working at the Central Texas VA [Veterans Administration] and facilitating a PTSD group. I was hearing stories from Vietnam veterans and other veterans and seeing how their experiences were still affecting them twenty, thirty, forty years later, to the point that when they were telling me stories they were breaking down in tears. That was the first time I'd ever been with a group that had been actually diagnosed with PTSD, they truly had it, and it just made it real to me. Some of them had turned to drugs and alcohol. Some had been financially ruined and lost their families. It made me hope that I would be deployed as a social worker on a combat stress control team in Iraq and then be able to go as far forward as possible. I thought if I could just be there when trauma happens and help people talk about it and bypass all that hurt, that would be better.

At the time I was sent to Tall Afar [an Iraqi city], it was extremely hot because it was close to the Syrian border and insurgents were coming over the border and taking over the town, almost like [the city of] Falluja. The Department of Defense decided it needed to get a whole regiment up there and take care of the city, clean it out, because voting was about to take place because it was December of '05. There was only a squadron—which is about eight hundred people—but about a week after I got there we learned that 3rd ACR [armored cavalry regiment] is all moving up, which is about five thousand soldiers. My unit was like, "Well, you're it, so take care of them." They came in and it was overwhelming to me. Luckily, because I had been in the army before, I was comfortable approaching commanders and asking for help in setting up shop.

Soldiers were going outside the wire [leaving the protection of their base] every day and I was probably there two weeks when I experienced my first day. It was late in the evening, about nine or ten o'clock, and I remember I was in the dining facility eating dinner, and one of the medics came and said, "We need your assistance at the TMC [troop medical clinic], a soldier has been shot." They brought him in on a tank and carried him into the troop medical clinic. He was shot by a sniper in Tall Afar. At that time it hit me that this is real, it's real. In that situation you just make yourself available in case the soldiers want to talk. The soldiers who carried the soldier into the camp were all distraught, very emotional. They were crying, bawling, wailing, and asking things like, "Why, why him?" Immediately I just felt helpless, seeing all these male soldiers just breaking down. I was just wondering, *What do I do?* Even the chaplain was wondering what to do. It was a platoon and they were using each other for support. The next day I introduced myself to the command and we arranged a critical-event debriefing. That was my first one.

Sadness, Grief, and Anger

Their feelings were a mix of sadness and grief and anger. They just experienced an insurgent killing not only their coworker but friend, so they were very angry. Why him? He was one of the better guys. He'd do anything for you. They would get into not only what happened at the incident and how they were feeling, but they would reflect on the soldier. It was just very emotional and touching for me. I feel very fortunate about what I experienced.

This was a bad event in the sense that the majority of the soldiers in his platoon witnessed it. It happened in a building that they were using for rest and recovery while they were in the city patrolling. They would go to this building and either take a nap or play cards. They had guards around the building, but the soldier was walking through the hallway to go down the steps, and through the window a sniper shot him and it hit him in his head. Soldiers witnessed this and they said it played as in slow motion. He fell to the ground and basically his head exploded, and they explained that the brains were all over the floor and there was gray matter and how it was so surreal, and then they went into further details and each one of them almost replayed it the same way and then shared how it affected them. I was amazed because I didn't think they would talk.

I did see him on the stretcher for a brief moment and then he was pronounced dead. That night when I went to sleep and a few nights after that I would shut my eyes and I would get a visual of what they explained. I would get all teary-eyed and ask myself, "Why are we here? Why do soldiers have to die like this? What's the purpose?" I just started questioning myself. It affected me pretty hard.

The chaplain and I used to talk to each other. When you do a critical-event debriefing the rule is to always have two people there; so he felt comfortable with conducting critical-event debriefings, so we would do them together, and after each critical-event debriefing we would debrief ourselves.

I think we had roughly thirty of those debriefings and I would say about twenty-two of them involved death or the death of a soldier. The other ones were for extreme traumatic events. There were quite a few suicide bombings in Tall Afar. Soldiers weren't injured, because suicide bombers were targeting people that were going to sign up to be a part of their police force or people going to vote, but there were mass suicide bombings where thirty or more people were killed. The soldiers had to witness it and clean up the aftermath. Part of our mission is humanitarian, so we clean that up, we package up the bodies as best we can and send them basically to the mortuary. That was one of the soldiers' tasks. Could you imagine being an eighteen-year-old private and having to go clean up thirty bodies that were just blown apart, picking up an arm here, a leg there, and putting arms in a pile and legs in a pile, then trying to figure out what goes with what body? It's extremely traumatic. The biggest concern soldiers had was seeing the children. Children were blown so high that they would land on the roofs of buildings, and soldiers had to go and retrieve the bodies. They said that really affected them, mostly because they had children of their own.

Some soldiers would come and talk to me and be fearful that, yes, they didn't know what to expect, especially with the threat of IEDs [improvised explosive devices]. They can be anywhere, and they can be remotely detonated. The first, lead vehicle could go over an IED and the second thinks this is a clear path, but there is someone over there with a remote control and as soon as the second vehicle goes over, it is detonated. The whole unknowing aspect of what's going to happen when they leave the wire is what soldiers were fearful of. They accepted the fact that every time they went outside the wire they could potentially get killed, but their fear was, Well, what if I don't get killed and I just lose my arm, I couldn't make it through life with a handicap.

Fear of Doing the Wrong Thing

Being away from their families was a big stressor for them. The fear of maybe doing the wrong thing with all the chaos that's over there and our rules of engagement always changing—they were fearful that they would get put in a situation where they would have to decide, "Should I fire my weapon to save my buddy, or if I fire my weapon and kill this person am I going to get prosecuted because I didn't follow the rules of engagement?"

Unfortunately, I had a soldier who was on a mission and part of his mission was to ensure that vehicles were not going to be driving down a certain roadway, and he fired his weapon because the Iraqis weren't halting and he did kill two children. That was very traumatic for him and he was a young guy who had children of his own. The fact that he took two children's lives was very hard for him, even though his platoon buddies reassured him he did the right thing. He was not charged with anything. It was just a tragedy of war.

On occasion, as a mental health professional, I do have a conflict of interest about doing my clients, the soldiers, the least amount of harm. There were a lot of cases where my professional opinion was ... that this soldier was in Iraq during the first rotation, redeployed back to the U.S. where he was appropriately diagnosed with PTSD, getting treatment with medication and individual therapy, but due to the need, he is cleared to go back for a second tour. Clearly this just adds to his symptoms. The DSM [Diagnostic and Statistical Manual] has actually come out with a new definition of that kind of PTSD, where it accumulates, called complex PTSD. I've already seen problems with the redeployment of soldiers. This one soldier was on his second deployment, and he talked to me about how the first time was bad and he was appropriately diagnosed with PTSD, but this time around he knows he is adding to his issues, even though he was getting through it. I believe there are many soldiers out there in the same situation. They are coping and able to do their job, but in the long run I think it is going to hit them overwhelmingly.

At my level, all I can do is recommend they go for evaluation. Under the Department of Defense's standard, if it's not too extreme we give them rest and recoup time, let them vent a little bit. We give them some counseling and then put them back in their unit. If they can still function, they can stay there, but just because they can function, it doesn't mean that the continuation of experiencing trauma isn't going to hurt them in the long run. Maybe a month or ten years after they get back, this could hurt them more, so I did have an ethical dilemma with that, but unfortunately, that's not my call, you know, when you're a professional in the military.

The way I resolved it was to tell myself that it was beyond me. I was honest with soldiers and I explained to them that my professional opinion was, You're not doing so well, your sleep is off, your eating is off, you're obviously stressed, possibly depressed, but I encourage you to keep speaking with me about what's going on, to help cope with it through your time here. See a chaplain, talk to your buddies. I tell them, As soon as you get back home, go to mental health, get everything documented, because in the long run if you do get out of the army and you're still having issues, you need to turn to the VA and get help.

After seeing so many people, I started ordering stress balls and relaxation CDs and aromatherapy candles, self-help books, anything tangible I could give the soldiers to help them other than the counseling and the recommendations on things to do. I tried to get them to use any and every resource I could provide for them. Sometimes I would feel extremely helpless.

Chronology

1600s A.D.

Mental illness is regarded as God's punishment for sins committed by the individual or as evidence of demonic possession. The mentally ill are cared for at home or in poorhouses.

1692

Witchcraft is a common explanation for mental illness. In the Massachusetts Bay Colony, the Salem witchcraft trials sentenced nineteen people to hanging.

1724

Puritan clergyman Cotton Mather sees evidence of the workings of Divine Providence in the so-called distracted person but also writes that there might be physical explanations for mental illness.

1751

The Pennsylvania Hospital is founded by Dr. Thomas Bond and Benjamin Franklin "to care for the sick-poor and insane who were wandering the streets of Philadelphia."

1812

Benjamin Rush writes the first U.S. textbook on the subject of mental illness, *Medical Inquiries and Observations upon the Diseases of the Mind,* in which he describes madness as a disease.

1827

In New York State an "Act Concerning Lunatics" forbids the confinement of the mentally ill in prisons or houses of detention.

1833

Worcester State Lunatic Hospital opens in Worcester, Massachusetts. It is the first public asylum in the state.

1841

Reformer Dorothea Dix calls on the Massachusetts state legislature to care for the mentally ill, who are often kept in jails and prisons where they suffer physical abuse. Her efforts lead to the establishment of state mental hospitals.

1844

Under the leadership of Dr. Thomas Kirkbride, superintendents of asylums form the Association of Medical Superintendents of American Institutions for the Insane, the first national medical society in the nation. It later becomes the American Psychiatric Association.

1845

New Jersey State Hospital in Trenton is the first mental asylum to open following Kirkbride's plan of large, sprawling buildings situated on extensive plots of land. The concept is to promote privacy and comfort for the patients with the goal of hastening a cure.

1890

Under the New York State Care Act, the state assumes full responsibility for the mentally ill in the state.

1908

Neurologist and psychiatrist Adolf Meyer first uses the term "mental hygiene" to describe the maintenance of mental stability.

1909

The National Committee for Mental Hygiene is founded to advocate for improved care for the institutionalized mentally ill and for the prevention of mental illness.

1920s

State mental asylums are overcrowded with many kinds of patients, including the mentally ill, the poor and indigent, and the sick elderly.

1930s

Psychiatrists begin to use insulin to shock patients and place them in a temporary coma. It is used as a treatment for schizophrenia.

1936

Egas Moniz publishes an account of the first frontal lobotomy, a type of brain surgery used to treat mental illness that is later popularized in the United States by Dr. Walter Freeman.

1940s

Electroconvulsive therapy is first used in hospitals in the United States as a treatment for depression and other forms of mental illness.

1946

The Mental Health Act is passed by the federal government. It provides funding for research into the causes, prevention, and treatment of mental illness.

1947

Fountain House, in New York City, is established by former patients of Rockland State Hospital to serve as an activity and job-training center for the mentally ill. It becomes a model for other such "clubhouses" throughout the nation and in other countries.

1948

Albert Deutsch's book, *The Shame of the States*, exposes issues of overcrowding and neglect in America's state mental asylums.

1949

The National Institute of Mental Health (NIMH) is established under the Mental Health Act. NIMH becomes the federal government's leading agency on mental health issues.

1952

The first antipsychotic drug—chlorpromazine—is introduced to treat schizophrenics and others. Its widespread use (under the name Thorazine) enables many long-term patients to be released from hospitals.

1954

New York State enacts the Community Mental Health Services Act to provide state funds for outpatient clinics. Other states follow New York's model and expand community facilities.

1960s

The use of the drug lithium provides a breakthrough in the treatment of manic depression (now called bipolar disorder).

1963

The U.S. Congress passes laws intended to create Community Mental Health Centers (CMHCs) that will provide mental health treatment to all members of the community regardless of their ability to pay.

1965

Government policy aims to reduce the role of mental hospitals in favor of community care and treatment thus paving the way for the deinstitutionalization of many mentally ill persons. The passage of Medicaid in the same year leads to the transfer of elderly persons with mental disabilities from mental hospitals to nursing homes.

1970s

Deinstitutionalization—the process of releasing mental patients from state asylums into the community—results in widespread homelessness and neglect for many mentally ill patients. This is due to a lack of adequate outpatient treatment facilities, which were envisioned as the source of care that would allow the mentally ill to be rehabilitated and reintegrated into their communities.

1972

In the Supreme Court decision *Wyatt v. Stickney*, minimal standards are established for the adequate treatment of the mentally ill.

1972

A federal case in Wisconsin, *Lessard v. Schmidt*, leads to dramatic changes in the process of involuntarily committing someone for treatment in a mental institution. As a result of this case, people subject to commitment proceedings gain many of the rights accorded to criminal suspects, such as the right to counsel, and can only be committed if it is determined that they pose an imminent threat to themselves or others.

1979

The National Alliance for the Mentally Ill (NAMI) is formed to advocate for seriously mentally ill people and their families.

1986

The U.S. Congress authorizes the PAIMI program with the passage of the Protection and Advocacy for Individuals with Mental Illness Act. The program's goal is to protect and advocate for services to individuals with mental illness.

1998

The Treatment Advocacy Center (TAC) is founded to eliminate legal and clinical barriers to the timely and humane treatment of the mentally ill. TAC educates civic, legal, criminal justice, and legislative communities on the benefits of assisted treatment in an effort to decrease homelessness, jailings, suicide, violence, and other consequences of lack of treatment.

1999

In New York State, Kendra's law creates a framework for court-ordered assisted outpatient treatment for the mentally ill.

2002

According to the National Mental Health Association, at least twenty-nine states cut their mental health expenditures.

2006

A report issued by the National Association of State Mental Health Program Directors reveals that the mentally ill are dying on average twenty-five years earlier than the rest of the population.

2007

The Veterans Administration faces the mental health problems (such as post-traumatic stress disorder) of veterans returning from Afghanistan and Iraq.

Organizations to Contact

The editors compiled the following list of organizations con-cerned with the topics discussed in this book. The descriptions are from materials provided by the organizations. All have infor-mation available for interested readers. The list was compiled just prior to publication of the present volume; the information provided here may change. Be aware that many organizations take several weeks or longer to respond to inquiries, so allow as much time as possible.

American Psychological Association (APA)
750 First St. NE, Washington, DC   20002-4242
(800) 374-2721
Web site: www.apa.org

The APA provides information for professionals, students, and the general public about mental health issues. Its Web site in-cludes programs, affiliate organizations, conferences, informa-tion for consumers of mental health services, and information on a wide variety of mental health topics such as addiction, bipolar disorder, depression, PTSD, and schizophrenia. The site is updated every twenty-four hours.

Depression and Bipolar Support Alliance
730 N. Franklin St., Suite 501, Chicago, IL   60610-7224
(800) 826-3632 • fax: (312) 642-7243
Web site: www.dbsalliance.org

The Depression and Bipolar Support Alliance is a leading not-for-profit organization devoted to helping patients understand and manage their depression or bipolar disorder. It provides educational materials and scientific information written for the layperson, it runs programs, and it helps organize patient-run support groups. It also advocates for equal treatment for people with mood disorders.

Federation of Families for Children's Mental Health

9605 Medical Center Dr., Suite 280, Rockville, MD   20850
(240) 403-1901 • fax: (240) 403-1909
Web site: www.ffcmh.org

This national family-run organization advocates for the rights of children and youth with emotional, behavioral, and mental health issues and their families. It also works with federal, state, and local agencies and policy shapers to help advance the cause of children's mental health.

Mental Health America (MHA)

2000 N. Beauregard St., 6th Floor, Alexandria, VA   22311
(703) 684-7722 • fax: (703) 684-5968
Web site: www.mentalhealthamerica.net

Formerly known as the National Mental Health Association, Mental Health America is a nonprofit organization dedicated to helping people live mentally healthier lives. MHA has more than 320 affiliates across the United States. The affiliates are composed of individuals recovering from mental illness or addictions, families with mentally ill members, mental health-care professionals, advocates for mental health issues, researchers and others who work to educate the public about mental illness, fight for access to effective care, foster innovation in research, and promote mental wellness.

National Alliance on Mental Illness (NAMI)

2107 Wilson Blvd., Suite 300, Arlington, VA   22201-3042
(703) 524-7600 • fax: (703) 524-9094
Web site: www.nami.org

NAMI is the largest grassroots organization dedicated to helping improve the lives of the mentally ill and their families in the United States. It supports, educates, researches, and advocates on behalf of the mentally ill through its Web site, a toll-free helpline, and public awareness activities such as Mental Illness Awareness Week. Founded in 1979, NAMI serves as the umbrella organization for its local chapters in every state and in over one thousand communities.

National Alliance for Research on Schizophrenia and Depression (NARSAD)

60 Cutter Mill Rd., Suite 404, Great Neck, NY   11021-3196
(800) 829-8289 • fax: (516) 487-6930
Web site: www.narsad.org

NARSAD works to find cures for schizophrenia, depression, anxiety, and other mental diseases through donations and grants to scientists and scientific organizations. NARSAD-funded scientists use the latest innovations from the human genome project to explore the relationship between genes, the environment, and mental illness. The organization also provides individuals with information and news about the latest treatments for psychiatric diseases.

National Eating Disorders Association (NEDA)

603 Stewart St., Suite 803, Seattle, WA   98101
(800) 931-2237
Web site: www.edap.org

NEDA is the largest nonprofit organization in the nation devoted to preventing eating disorders. As part of its mission, NEDA provides treatment referrals to persons suffering from anorexia, bulimia, and binge-eating disorder as well as to those obsessed with body image and weight concerns. The goal of NEDA is the elimination of eating disorders through education, programs, and services.

National Institute of Mental Health (NIMH)

Public Information and Communications Branch
Bethesda, MD   20892-9663
(301) 443-4513 • fax: (301) 443-4279
Web site: www.nimh.nih.gov

NIMH is the lead federal agency for research on mental and behavioral disorders. It is one of twenty-seven components of the National Institutes of Health, the federal government's principal agency for biomedical and behavioral research. NIMH is involved in planning mental health initiatives and research into specific areas. It asks for information from patients, mental health advocates, scientists, Congress, the public and other mental health advocacy groups and disseminates this information to the government and public.

New York State Office of Mental Health (OMH)
44 Holland Ave., Albany, NY   12229
(800) 597-8481
Web site: www.omh.state.ny

New York State has one of the largest, most extensive mental health systems in the United States servicing more than five hundred thousand individuals each year. The OMH operates psychiatric centers and regulates, certifies, and oversees more than twenty-five hundred programs operated by towns and cities and by not-for-profit organizations. The programs include inpatient and outpatient programs, community support, and residential and family care programs.

Substance Abuse and Mental Health
Services Administration (SAMHSA)
National Mental Health Information Center
Washington, DC   20015
(800) 789-2647 • fax: (240) 221-4295
Web site: http://mentalhealth.samhsa.gov

SAMHSA is a U.S. federal agency that provides funding and support to community mental health and substance abuse treatment centers. Its National Mental Health Information Center was developed for users of mental health services and their families, the public, policy makers, health-care providers, and the media. It provides information about mental health through its toll-free telephone number, a Web site, and its publications. The staff at the information center directs callers to organizations that treat and prevent mental illness.

For Further Research

Books

Xavier Amador and Anna Lica, *I Am Not Sick, I Don't Need Help!* Peconic, NY: Vida, 2007.

Nancy Boyd-Franklin, *Black Families in Therapy: Understanding the African-American Experience.* New York: Guilford, 2003.

Daniel J. Flannery, *Violence and Mental Health in Everyday Life: Prevention and Intervention Strategies for Children and Adolescents.* Lanham, MD: AltaMira, 2006.

Lawrence J. Friedman, *Menninger: The Family and the Clinic.* New York: Knopf, 1990.

Lynn Gamwell and Nancy Tomes, *Madness in America: Cultural and Medical Perceptions of Mental Illness Before 1914.* Ithaca, NY: Cornell University Press, 1995.

Gerald N. Grob, *The Dilemma of Federal Mental Health Policy: Radical Reform or Incremental Change?* New Brunswick, NJ: Rutgers University Press, 2006.

Stephen Hinshaw, *The Mark of Shame: Stigma of Mental Illness and an Agenda for Change.* New York: Oxford University Press, 2007.

Tara Elgin Holley, *My Mother's Keeper: A Daughter's Memoir of Growing Up in the Shadow of Schizophrenia.* New York: HarperPerennial, 1998.

Ilona Meagher, *Moving a Nation to Care: Post-Traumatic Stress Disorder and America's Returning Troops.* Brooklyn, NY: Ig, 2007.

Margaret Muckenhoupt, *Dorothea Dix: Advocate for Mental Health Care.* New York: Oxford University Press, 2003.

Sylvia Nasar, *A Beautiful Mind: A Biography of John Forbes Nash Jr.* New York: Simon & Schuster, 1998.

Steven Noll and James W. Trent Jr., *Mental Retardation in America: A Historical Reader.* New York: New York University Press, 2004.

Susan Sheehan, *Is There No Place on Earth for Me?* New York: Random House, 1983.

Marie L. Thompson, *Mental Illness.* Westport, CT: Greenwood, 2007.

E. Fuller Torrey, *Surviving Schizophrenia: A Manual for Families, Consumers, and Providers.* New York: Harper-Perennial, 1995.

Rogers H. Wright and Nicholas Cummings, *Destructive Trends in Mental Health: The Well-Intentioned Path to Harm.* London: Routledge, 2005.

Periodicals

Julian E. Barnes, "Repeat Duty Tied to Acute Stress," *Los Angeles Times*, December 20, 2006.

Bruce Bower, "Immigration Blues," *Science News*, December 18, 2004.

Marilyn Elias, "Job, Family Counseling Key to Schizophrenics' Independence," *USA Today*, March 1, 2007.

Chris L. Jenkins, "A Painful Choice over the Mentally Disabled," *Washington Post*, December 19, 2006.

Barbara Kantrowitz, "'I Never Knew What to Expect'; Depressed Parents Often Leave Their Children a Legacy of Fear and Anxiety," *Newsweek*, February 26, 2007.

Vikram Patel, "Mental Health Matters," *New Scientist*, August 21, 2004.

Richard Perez-Peña, "Law Says Insurers Must Pay for Care of the Mentally Ill," *New York Times*, December 23, 2006.

Patrick Perry, "Jane Pauley: Tackling the Stigma of Bipolar Disorder," *Saturday Evening Post*, March/April 2007.

Lee Romney and Scott Gold, "Breakdown; Tragedy Follows Landmark Court Win," *Los Angeles Times*, March 16, 2007.

Mary Ellen Schneider, "Better Coordination of Mental, Physical Health Urged," *Clinical Psychiatry News*, February 2007.

Chris Sigurdson, "The Mad, the Bad and the Abandoned: The Mentally Ill in Prisons and Jails," *Corrections Today*, December 2000.

Internet Sources

"Mental Health: Promise Unfulfilled," *Governing.com*, February 2004. www.governing.com/gpp/2004/mental.htm.

Bengt Jansson, "Controversial Psychosurgery Resulted in a Nobel Prize," *Nobelprize.org*, October 29, 1998. http://nobelprize.org/nobel_prizes/medicine/articles/moniz/index.html.

Mental Health America, "Position Statement 58: Health and Wellness for People with Serious Mental Illness." www.nmha.org/goposition-statements/p-58.

National Public Radio, "Military Mental Health Care Under Scrutiny," *All Things Considered*, March 6, 2007. www.npr.org/templates/story/story.php?storyId=7738485&ft=1&f=1003.

Office of the U.S. Surgeon General, "Mental Health: A Report of the Surgeon General." www.surgeongeneral.gov/library/mentalhealth/home.html.

Psychiatric Services, "Gold Award: The Wellspring of the Clubhouse Model for Social and Vocational Adjustment of Persons with Serious Mental Illness," November 1999. http://psychservices.psychiatryonline.org/cgi/content/full/50/11/1473.

Public Broadcasting Service, "Mentally Ill Homeless," January 3, 2003. www.pbs.org/religionandethics/week618/cover.html.

Sound Portraits.org, "My Lobotomy," http://soundportraits.org/on-air/my_lobotomy/.

Jamie Tolan, "Rustic Dreams, Human Nightmares," *Newsday.com*, www.newsday.com/community/guide/lihistory/ny-century_of_science_dispsych,0,4727264.story?coll=ny-lihistory-navigation.

Index

W

War exhaustion. *See* Post-
  traumatic stress disorder (PTSD)
Ward, Mary Jane, 140
Warham, John, 39
Warning out, 33–34
Welfare system and care, 180
Whitaker, Robert, 42
Williams, Anthony, 173
Williams, G. Mennen, 141
Winkelman, William, 120
Witchcraft, 36, 38, 215

Women Iraq War veterans, 16
Wood, Trish, 208
Worcester State Lunatic Hospital
  (MA), 216
Workhouses, 25
Wyatt v. Stickney, 219

Y

Yonkman, F. F., 122

Z

Zander, Tom, 165